Praise for *Chakras for Creativity*

"Inspiring and informative, *Chakras for Creativity* is a treasure ~~chest of exercises guar~~anteed to get your creative juices flowing … I'll be keeping this book on my desk so I can reach for it when I'm in need of a boost." **—Sally-Anne Lomas, artist, filmmaker, and author of *Live Like Your Head's on Fire***

"Whether you are an experienced yogi or someone who is looking to be inspired, this book will give you the tools to unblock energy and allow your creative juices to flow." **—Donna Negus, yoga and mindfulness teacher**

"When Jilly writes a book, there comes a calm, confident, and friendly guiding hand and heart. She takes us deeper into an area, an interest, a way of life. This latest offering … will be a delight and an ongoing source of reference to yoga students and teachers alike." **—Lindsey Porter, Yoga Scotland yoga tutor, author of *Whirlpools, Yoga and the Balance of Life***

"A welcome addition to the bookshelf on creativity especially for those who prefer a physical approach." **—Bethany Rivers, author of *Fountain of Creativity* and editor of *As Above So Below* online poetry magazine**

"The contents, although profound, are very accessible and will be of great benefit to teachers and practitioners of both yoga and mindfulness as well as to creative people who may be struggling to give birth to new ideas … A generous, wise, and deeply helpful book." **—Marilyn Buckham, yoga and mindfulness teacher**

"Bespoke asana sequences, walking and writing meditations, sound, mantras, colors and mandalas all combine in an accessible, practical way, helping us tap into the transformational power of these seven wheels of energy." **—Judy Brenan, British Wheel of Yoga teacher**

"Once I started to read this book, I couldn't put it down…When I then entered my studio, I was able to simply let go and dance with my imagination. Paintings that were not finished were suddenly being completed … A must-read for anyone who wants to really blossom into their full creative potential." **—Ian Baker Johnson, artist and life coach**

"*Chakras for Creativity* is certainly not 'just another book about chakras'… This book contains an extensive explanation of the chakra system from ancient texts, but its impact comes from the imaginative way that everyone can unlock their true creative potential." —**Clare Badham, yoga teacher**

"A treasure trove of varied, rich, and magical practice which will unlock the potential of every reader one petal at a time… This book should come with a warning: Be aware, *Chakras for Creativity* will have an enduringly positive impact on your health, well-being, and creativity." —**Angela Ripley co-founder of Om Yoga Works and Om Yoga Works Foundation**

"Every page spills over with wisdom… This charming, friendly book will help anyone use the chakra model to better know themselves… This is one to read straight through at first encounter, then revisit time and time again." —**Sage Rountree, PhD, E-RYT 500, author of *Everyday Yoga* and *Teaching Yoga Beyond the Poses***

"Mapping through the body from earth to sky, Jilly presents a range of techniques, tools, and activities that are simple and yet very effective in accessing one's own unique creative potential, empowerment, and expression." —**Jean Hall, yoga teacher and author of *Breathe***

"Jilly presents a clear, fresh perspective on the chakras, just what you would expect from a creativity-based book. This is a brilliant, go-to guide for everyone who wants to develop their creative gifts and abilities… It is beautifully written and organized in an easy-to-follow manner. Highly recommended." —**Julie Lusk, author of *Yoga Nidra Meditations***

CHAKRAS
FOR CREATIVITY

About the Author

Jilly Shipway is the author of *Yoga Through the Year* and *Yoga by the Stars*. She is a qualified yoga teacher and has more than thirty years of teaching experience. Over her long teaching career, she has enthused hundreds of students with her love of yoga, and many of them have continued to study with her for many years and up to the present day. She has tutored foundation-level, pre-diploma yoga study courses for the British Wheel of Yoga. Jilly was fortunate to have discovered yoga in her early teens and so has had a lifetime of studying and practicing yoga.

Jilly has been studying the chakras and integrating chakra-inspired yoga practices into her own home practice and her yoga classes and courses for over twenty years. In this book, *Chakras for Creativity*, Jilly shares the tried and tested techniques that have helped her overcome many challenges in her life and have supercharged her own creativity. She has developed a uniquely imaginative and practical approach to yoga, and she is passionate to share it with others through her teaching and writing.

Jilly has a BA (Hons) in fine art. After finishing art college, she worked for several years as an art and craft instructor for children and for adults with learning difficulties. Much of the artwork in this and her other two books is based on Jilly's original artwork.

As well as teaching general yoga classes, she also has many years of experience teaching specialist yoga classes to adults recovering from mental health problems. She trained at King's College London as a motivational interviewing coach, coaching people caring for someone with an eating disorder, and worked under the supervision of Professor Janet Treasure and her team.

Jilly regularly contributes to various magazines and publications, including *The Yoga Magazine*, *Spirit and Destiny* magazine, *Llewellyn's Witches' Datebook*, and the *Llewellyn's Moon Sign Book*.

When she is not teaching, writing about, or doing yoga, she loves walking, being in nature, and connecting with family and friends. She lives in the UK in a small Welsh border town, surrounded by hills. She is married and has one grown-up daughter.

Visit her websites at www.yogabythestars.com and www.chakrasforcreativity.com.

CHAKRAS
FOR CREATIVITY

Meditations & Yoga-Based Practices
to Awaken Your Creative Potential

JILLY SHIPWAY

Llewellyn Publications
Woodbury, Minnesota

FIRST EDITION
First Printing, 2022

Book design by Christine Ha
Cover design by Cassie Willett
Interior art
  Caduceus symbol (page 19) & chakra symbols (pages 57, 75, 91, 111, 129, 145 & 161) by the Llewellyn Art Department
  Chakra figure (page 23) by Mary Ann Zapalac
  Interior yoga illustrations by Llewellyn Art Department, based on art by Jilly Shipway

Llewellyn Publications is a registered trademark of Llewellyn Worldwide Ltd.

Library of Congress Cataloging-in-Publication Data
Names: Shipway, Jilly, author.
Title: Chakras for creativity : meditations & yoga-based practices to awaken your creative potential / Jilly Shipway.
Description: First edition. | Woodbury, Minnesota : Llewellyn Publication, 2022. | Includes bibliographical references. | Summary: "Through yoga, meditation, and visualization exercises, Jilly Shipway shows you how to tap into your chakras and enhance your creativity. Working with these seven energy centers can help you bring more success into all areas of your life, including art projects, business endeavors, scientific pursuits, and more"— Provided by publisher.
Identifiers: LCCN 2022037577 (print) | LCCN 2022037578 (ebook) | ISBN 9780738772783 (paperback) | ISBN 9780738773247 (ebook)
Subjects: LCSH: Chakras. | Yoga. | Meditations.
Classification: LCC BF1442.C53 S5443 2022 (print) | LCC BF1442.C53 (ebook) | DDC 294.5/43—dc23/eng/20220824
LC record available at https://lccn.loc.gov/2022037577
LC ebook record available at https://lccn.loc.gov/2022037578

Llewellyn Worldwide Ltd. does not participate in, endorse, or have any authority or responsibility concerning private business transactions between our authors and the public.
  All mail addressed to the author is forwarded, but the publisher cannot, unless specifically instructed by the author, give out an address or phone number.
  Any internet references contained in this work are current at publication time, but the publisher cannot guarantee that a specific location will continue to be maintained. Please refer to the publisher's website for links to authors' websites and other sources.

Llewellyn Publications
A Division of Llewellyn Worldwide Ltd.
2143 Wooddale Drive
Woodbury, MN 55125-2989
www.llewellyn.com

Printed in the United States of America

For Ada Mary, my grandmother.
Thank you for igniting my creative spark.

Disclaimer

CONTENTS

EXERCISES

Yoga Practices

Chakra Meditations and Visualizations

Chakra Walking Meditations

Chakra Writing Meditations

Chakra Meditation Questions

ACKNOWLEDGMENTS

A book is always a team effort, and, once again, it has been a pleasure to collaborate with the production team at Llewellyn Worldwide, who have worked so hard to make this book the best it can be. I owe a huge debt of gratitude to my wonderful editor, Angela Wix, for her impeccable judgment, and for guiding me so expertly through three books now! Also, a big thank you to my production editor, Lauryn Heineman, for her painstaking work and for always being a pleasure to work with. Thanks also to Aundrea Foster, copywriter; Cassie Willett, cover designer; and Christine Ha, production designer.

Thank you to my husband, Simon. Your love, support, and encouragement mean so much to me! Thank you to Kay, my daughter, who is one of the most creative people I know, and the seed of the idea for this book grew from our conversations about creativity.

Thank you to Natalie Goldberg, whose teachings and writing inspired me, many years ago, to commit to cultivating writing as a meditation. And to Thich Nhat Hanh for his teachings and writing that always remind me to walk meditatively and even on the darkest day to look up and enjoy the beauty of the sky.

Thank you to Anodea Judith for her groundbreaking work, which has expanded and enriched our understanding of the chakras.

My own yoga practice, teaching, and writing have been enriched by the inspirational teachings of Vanda Scaravelli, Sandra Sabatini, Donna Farhi, Judith Lasater, Cyndi Lee, Sarah Powers, Erich Schiffmann, and Gary Kraftsow.

I am grateful to Julie Lusk for writerly support and encouragement; to Summer Cushman for her radical, loving, and authentic approach to yoga; and to Judy Brenan for friendship, support, and great conversations about yoga!

Thank you to all the students who have studied yoga with me over the years. I have learned so much from teaching you, and your invaluable feedback. Especial thanks to my regular yoga classes, who every week bring sunshine into my life!

Thank you to Helen and Steve Collins for fun, games, and laughter! Libby James for love and encouragement. The walkers' group for walking, talking, and great cake stops! To Alison Ash for loving and challenging conversations and for being a great friend. And thanks to Amie Allen, osteopath, for helping me to stay balanced and aligned during the process of writing this book.

And finally, thank you to that creative spark within us all that prompts us to reimagine the world and expand our sense of what is possible through our wild, messy, and beautiful creativity!

And if you fall in love with the imagination,
you understand that it is a free spirit.
It will go anywhere, do anything.

—Alice Walker

INTRODUCTION

Ignite Your Creative Spark!

Young children view the world through the prism of a rainbow. Everything is new to them. The question that is continually on their lips is "Why?" They have a sense of wonder. They are playful. The world is full of possibilities. They learn through play. Their world is not fixed. What happens along the way to make us forget that we once saw the world as a magical place, full of infinite possibilities? Why does life become humdrum, and we slip into autopilot and stop seeing the beauty and potential all around us? Imagination is like a muscle, and when not used, it grows weak and atrophies.

To live a creative life, we must start to see the world through fresh eyes, no longer blindly accepting that this is just the way things are and instead asking ourselves, how could things be done differently? When the first astronauts looked down on Earth, suspended in the dark emptiness of space, the realization of Earth's beauty and fragility dawned on them with crystal-clarity. Although we might not get to fly to the moon, we can change our perspective and look at the world from a different angle. Now more than ever, when we live in a world burdened with so many potentially catastrophic problems, we need the power of creative minds to generate lifesaving solutions. We also look to creativity and yoga to give us respite, relaxation, and refuge from the stresses caused by living through such turbulent times.

The creative person uses her imagination to generate ideas. She problem-solves. She invents. She creates. Creativity is when you are faced with an impossible situation, and yet each morning you get up and say, "I can find a way through this." And although you can't yet see the light at the end of the tunnel, in your mind's eye you can picture that light, and you are heading toward it. Creativity is when you love yourself despite all of society's messages that you are unworthy of love. This radical love is creativity.

Sadly, many people have bad experiences in their formative years that convince them that they are not creative. When I left art college in the early 1980s, I worked for a year in a primary school, each day working with a different class and doing art with them. I clearly remember one teacher shouting at a five-year-old girl because the girl had given the person in her drawing blue hair. "What color is hair?" the teacher shouted at the wide-eyed child. "It certainly is not blue!" This teacher had evidently never seen a Picasso painting during his blue phase. It is the sort of event that can put a child off drawing for life and convince them that they can't draw. It is much more helpful to simply ask a child to tell you about their drawing. The colors they use may not be a photographic representation of a real person, but they allow the child to express what they are feeling. Drawing is often used as therapy for children who have suffered traumatic experiences such as war.

I remember, aged five years old, on my first day at school, being given a handful of colored crayons and a black and white line drawing of an apple to color in. I was happily drawing away when the teaching assistant gently reprimanded me for not coloring in within the lines. She patiently showed me how to color in and not go over the black outline. It was a good skill to learn, but one that as a young adult studying art I had to unlearn. Sometimes it's good to stay within the lines; at other times what's needed is to allow the paint to flow freely across your page or canvas. By the time that I was sitting at a table and drawing with my own young daughter, there were fabulous coloring books available called anti-coloring books that encouraged children (and adults!) to let their imagination run wild.

Fortunately, although our creative confidence can be dented by negative childhood experiences, the human spirit is resilient, and the creative impulse is not easily extinguished. This is fortunate because there are so many proven benefits of creativity, which we will explore in more depth in part 1 of the book. The ancient yoga text the *Chandogya Upanishad* tells us that "there is a Light that shines beyond all things on earth, beyond us all, beyond the heaven, beyond the highest, the very highest heavens. This is the light that shines in our heart."[1] The purpose of this book is to help you to reconnect with the divine spark within you so that you can create magic in your life and fulfill your creative potential.

Of course, sometimes in life we go off track, losing our way, and at these times it feels like we have lost touch with our guiding light; we find ourselves wandering lost at the periphery of our life. Life becomes humdrum and we operate on autopilot, seeing the world in monochrome, rather than its spectrum of rainbow colors. The divine spark within each of us is like the flame of a candle seen through the glass of a lantern. If the glass gets dirty, then the flame of the candle will appear dim. However, once we have polished the glass, then the flame will once again shine brightly. The flame is constant and always there, resplendent in our heart space; it's just that the glass is soiled, and so the flame appears dim. Yoga shows us how to polish our metaphorical lantern, and then we are able, once again, to radiate our light out into the world.

This book is for you if you struggle with life (and who doesn't?), and yet you still want to sing your song, share your poem, write a story, make a protest banner, bake a cake, make up a bedtime story for your child, paint a picture, make love, knit a rainbow-colored jumper, or sew a friendship quilt. This book is for you if you are a person who wants to create beauty and share it with the world, even if sometimes your creative urges get submerged and buried deep under the minutiae of everyday life. Despite feeling overwhelmed, you still yearn to get creative and make life come alive again. This book is for you if you've always had the idea that you would like to do something creative, but you haven't gotten around to it yet, and you feel that there is a novel, symphony, painting, or some other masterpiece within you waiting to be released!

Chakras for Creativity

In this book I will outline chakra theory, but mainly as it relates to boosting your creative potential. I will also share with you many practical ways of using yoga, meditation, and visualizations so that you can directly experience the chakras and integrate their transformational power into your own creative path.

Traditionally, it is the second, sacral chakra that is considered to pertain most strongly to creativity, and this is most likely due to its association with water and the moon and its sensual relationship to pleasure, sexuality, and the creation of new life. However, to maximize our creative potential we must take a holistic approach to the chakras, as each one of

---

1. Juan Mascaro, trans., *The Upanishads* (London: Penguin, 1965), 113.

them supports and enhances our creativity in different but equally important ways, as the following list demonstrates:

Root Chakra: This blood-red chakra provides a solid foundation for your creativity. When you work with this chakra, you learn to take care of your basic survival needs, which leaves you free to build up your creativity from a secure and solid base. With the earth supporting you, you can put down roots and your creativity can grow and be sustained. This is the place where your creativity finds a home.

Sacral Chakra: Working with this watery chakra teaches you to ride the ebb and flow of your creativity. This juicy, orange chakra picks you up and carries you on a wave of pleasure and through your creativity you get to share that pleasure with others. The sacral chakra links your creativity to the umbilical cord of life, you learn about the attraction of opposites, and your ideas are fertilized and grow.

Solar Plexus Chakra: This chakra empowers you to radiate your creative light out into the world. It gives you the confidence to shine! Working with this chakra helps you develop an ability to take up creative space in the world. It fires up your creativity, and you find the will, the push, and the drive to get your creations out into the world.

Heart Chakra: This chakra breathes life and love into your creations. It helps you find a point of equilibrium between heaven and earth, resulting in your creations being harmonious and balanced. Working with this chakra teaches you to show compassion and love to yourself and others as you tread the creative path.

Communication Chakra: This chakra enables you to give voice to your creations and to communicate your vision. It teaches you to speak up and be heard but also to listen and learn. Working with this chakra teaches you to speak from the heart, to impart your wisdom through your creativity, and to receive wisdom through creative listening.

Third Eye Chakra: Working with this chakra develops your intuition, clairvoyance, and imagination. You learn to see with your inner eye, to visualize what it is you wish to create, and to recall your dreams and be guided by them. Your creative vision is illuminated, and you are open to receiving inspiration from above. You see and you know.

Crown Chakra: Working with this chakra is transformative. It releases your inner spark of genius, and you relax into a state of pure bliss. You are now able to rise above everyday concerns and connect with the sacred, and you are imbued with a sense of being at one with it all. You see the bigger picture and are no longer bogged down by the minutiae of life. You feel connected to the cosmos and open to receiving divine inspiration. Now you can see the celestial within the commonplace. Dive deep and uncover your creative gold!

We'll dive deeper into chakra wisdom in part 1, but for now, I hope the list gives you a taste of the ways that working with the seven chakras can support, nurture, nourish, and exponentially expand your creative potential.

Blossom into Your Creative Potential

I discovered and fell head over heels in love with yoga in my early teens, and so I have had a lifetime of studying and practicing yoga. In my twenties I trained to teach yoga, and I now have more than thirty years of teaching experience. I've been privileged to witness, over several decades, how my students, when working with the methods outlined in this book, blossom into their full creative potential.

For me, creativity and yoga have always gone hand in hand. My four years at art college, studying fine art to degree level, helped me develop a playful, creative, open-minded approach, which has stood me in good stead when designing creative and imaginative yoga practices. And the many years I spent in life-drawing classes, studying the naked human form, means that I draw exceptionally good yoga pin-people!

My impulse to write this book came from a desire to share the yoga and mindfulness techniques that have helped me overcome many challenges in my life and realize my dream of becoming a published yoga author. All the techniques I share with you in this book have been successfully integrated into my life, my yoga practice, and my teaching over decades. I know from experience that they work, and I know they have the power to transform your life and supercharge your creativity.

The Chakras for Creativity approach that I will be sharing with you in the book includes chakra meditations, yoga practices inspired by the chakras, walking meditations, writing meditations, and meditation questions. These techniques, which are simple to learn, will give you access to a treasure trove of creativity, and with regular practice they will allow you to access a deep source of inner wisdom that is the source of all creativity.

The yoga and mindfulness techniques described in the book are simple, effective, accessible, and short enough to easily be fitted into a busy life. Regardless of whether you are a professional creative or someone who wants to use creativity in your spare time to promote a sense of well-being, the practices in this book will benefit you. If you are a writer looking for ways to overcome writer's block, this book will show you ways to embrace, understand, and push through the block and, in the process, open yourself to a limitless source of inspiration. Whatever artistic field you are involved in, the practices will get your creative juices flowing again. Of course, creativity is not limited to the arts, and there are innumerable benefits from bringing a blue sky, open-minded, creative approach to business, the sciences, and everyday life generally. So whether you are a scientist, an artist, a chef, a mathematician, a dancer, or an environmental activist, you can benefit from strengthening your creative muscles.

How to Use This Book

This section will give you some tips on how to get the most out of this book and how to navigate your way around it. After you've read this section, move on to part 1, "The Chakras for Creativity Approach," where you'll learn more about the elements that are found in each of the chakra chapters and how best to work with them.

Each of the seven chakra chapters contains the following elements:

- A chakra at-a-glance guide
- An introduction to the chakra
- A guide to yoga inspired by the chakra
- A chakra-inspired yoga practice
- A chakra meditation or visualization
- A chakra walking meditation
- Chakra writing meditations ideas
- A set of chakra meditation questions

After you have read part 1, you're ready to dive into the chakra chapters in part 2. First time around, I'd suggest that you begin at the root chakra chapter and work your way through the book to the crown chakra chapter. This will give you a really good foundational understanding of the seven chakras and how to work with them to boost your creativity. After that, you're good to dip into the chakra chapters in any way that works for you.

As you gain more experience working with the chakras, you'll find you intuitively know which chakra you need to pay more attention to. I expect you'll return to the book at various times and for different reasons. Most of us need to regularly work on the root chakra to ensure that we have strong foundations, stability, and support in our lives. Or, for example, if you're feeling creatively blocked, revisiting the sacral chakra chapter will get your creativity flowing again. When you're in need of being assertive go to the solar plexus chakra. For a rigid attitude, try reconnecting with your loving heart chakra. To find your voice, go to the communication chakra. To boost imagination and insight, go to the third eye chakra chapter. And to bring more blissful "simply being" moments into your life, go to the crown chakra chapter.

This book is a practical guide to the chakras, so reading the chakra chapters is your first step; however, it is by doing the chakra exercises in each chapter that you'll unlock the door to the extraordinary creative potential of the chakras. It is by practicing the chakra meditations, yoga, walking, writing, and meditation questions that you will gain access to the magical, transformative, bliss-inducing powers of the chakras!

I'm sure that as a creative person you will find your own innovative ways of using this book. Each time you read one of the chakra chapters and work with the exercises you are shining the light of your awareness onto that chakra and breathing life into it. This book is here as a lantern, shining a light on the path that leads to your creative fulfillment.

Now you're all set to move on to part 1 of the book, where we will explore the five main elements that make up the Chakras for Creativity approach.

PART I

The Chakras for Creativity Approach

CHAPTER 1
Yoga: The Mother of Invention

The Chakras for Creativity approach, outlined in this book, is a prayerful one. However, be reassured that this prayerful approach is beneficial and suitable for those of all religions or none. By "prayerful," what I mean is that we quieten down and open ourselves to guidance and creative inspiration. It is up to you to decide whether the guidance that you receive in the silence of contemplation comes from a divine source or from your own inner wisdom.

The mother origins of yoga can provide us with the basis for this prayerful, or contemplative, approach. According to Hindu tradition, the body of knowledge that we call *yoga* was born from the womb of the Earth itself.[2] And although Patanjali is often referred to as the "father" of yoga, it's less well known that his knowledge of yoga, which was organized by him into the Yoga Sutra, was handed down to him by his mother, Gonika. The story goes that in ancient times a wise yogini called Gonika was entrusted with passing on the ancient wisdom of yoga that the Earth had given birth to, ensuring that this sacred knowledge was preserved for future generations. For many years Gonika searched unsuccessfully for a suitable student to pass her knowledge on to. Finally, one

---

2. Georg Feuerstein, *The Yoga Tradition: Its History, Literature, Philosophy and Practice* (Prescott, AZ: Hohm Press, 2001), 214.

day as she stood by a waterfall that flowed into a river, she scooped up a handful of water into her cupped hands and prayed to the Sun God, saying, "This knowledge has come through you; let me give it back to you." The Sun God smiled down upon her and answered her prayer by dropping into her praying hands a serpent that had fallen from heaven, and she called him Patanjali. *Pata* means both "serpent" and "fallen"; *anjali* is the worshipful gesture of cupped hands.[3]

It can be helpful and inspiring to evoke the wisdom of Gonika at the start of a creative project or anytime you feel creatively blocked, so as to get your ideas flowing again. It will help you feel connected to a universal source of inspiration that is always available whenever you need a creative boost. To evoke the wisdom of Gonika, imagine that, like Gonika, you are standing by a waterfall that flows into a river, and raise your hands in prayer asking that creative wisdom may flow through you and back out into the world from whence it came. The water represents a fountain of creative ideas that is being constantly replenished. If it feels right, silently say, *This knowledge has come through you; let me give it back to you.* The idea behind this is that there is a circular flow of inspiration that we are tapping into, receiving, and then giving it back again to the source.

As stated earlier, this approach can be used in either a religious or a secular way. If you have religious beliefs, then during the visualization you might think of yourself tapping into knowledge from a divine source. If you are not of a religious disposition, you might want to visualize the knowledge or inspiration as coming from nature and being given back to her. Or alternatively, you might envision it as tapping into the source of your own inner wisdom, and it is that which is flowing through you and inspiring you.

In the Chakras for Creativity approach, we begin with a prayerful quietening down so that we might open ourselves up to receiving inspiration. This involves a period of quietening down, relaxing, focusing, and deep listening. However, once we are inspired, we act, we create, we manifest our vision in the world. We receive divine inspiration, and we give it back by creating beauty in the world.

Yoga and Creativity to Boost Well-Being

In truth the Path of Yoga and the Path of Creativity are not separate paths: they are one and the same. Linda Naiman, founder of Creativity at Work, says, "Creativity is the act of turning new and imaginative ideas into reality. Creativity is characterized by the ability to perceive the world in new ways, to find hidden patterns, to make connections

---

3. B. K. S. Iyengar, *The Tree of Yoga* (London: Thorsons, 2000), 74.

between seemingly unrelated phenomena, and to generate solutions."[4] Yoga, like creativity, seeks to unite complementary opposites with the goal of balancing these complementary opposites to reach a state of equilibrium and peace. In this state we feel a sense of unity and connection with all that is. The word *yoga* comes from Sanskrit, the scriptural language of ancient India. Its root is the verb *yuj*, meaning "to yoke" or "to unite." When we form a union between yoga and creativity, we set ourselves on a path that leads us on a lifelong journey toward wholeness.

Creativity, like yoga, has physical, emotional, and mental health benefits. Research has shown that engaging in creative activities improves mental and physical health, increases happiness, improves mood, and increases brain function.[5] Yoga's health benefits are well documented. In general terms physical yoga practice improves suppleness, flexibility, and strength. This means that because your body is functioning well, it frees you up to concentrate on getting on with life, including your creative endeavors, unimpeded by aches and pains.

Yoga practice, particularly working with the chakras, removes blockages that prevent your vital energy, *prana*, from flowing freely. Once your vital energy is circulating freely again, you will feel revitalized, energized, and open to receiving inspiration. Regular yoga practice helps us develop focus and concentration. We train ourselves to observe our thoughts and to come back to a single focus; this focused concentration means that we are more productive and less prone to distractions when we are involved in creative endeavors. Yogic states of relaxation and meditation improve clarity and self-knowledge and we develop trust in our inner wisdom, which leads us to being receptive to wild and wonderful creative ideas when they come to visit!

Both creativity and yoga are associated with rapturous states. Yogis believe that our natural state is one of bliss (*samadhi*). Likewise, artists talk of the rapture of being in the flow of the creative process. Sports people refer to it as "being in the zone." Bliss is a state of grace experienced by both yoga practitioners and those involved in creative endeavors. We can't "achieve" grace—it's not an endpoint. However, this book will share with you practices that will help you to create the right conditions for grace to unfold.

---

4. Linda Naiman, "What Is Creativity (And Why Is It Crucial for Business Success?)," Creativity at Work, last modified November 18, 2021, https://www.creativityatwork.com/what-is-creativity/.

5. Marcella McEvoy, "How Creativity and Hobbies Can Benefit Your Health," Bupa, February 20, 2020, https://www.bupa.co.uk/newsroom/ourviews/creativity-hobbies-benefit-health.

The state of yoga is one of bliss. When you enter that state, you feel a sense of union with all that is. This is not a state of doing; it is a state of being. You may have been fortunate enough already to have had a glimpse of this blissful state in your yoga practice or while fully absorbed in another activity, such as painting, writing, gardening, spending time in nature, making love, or making a fruit cake! Perhaps you have experienced it when walking in a beautiful landscape. The rhythm of your walking, the sun on your face, a view from the top of the mountain, and all at once, you no longer felt separate from your surroundings—you were part of it all.

Many yoga practitioners find that their most creative ideas arise from this yogic state of bliss. Author Julie Lusk found that the entire concept for her wonderful book *Yoga Nidra Meditations* came to her during a yoga nidra session. Likewise, I often find that the answer to a creative problem that I have been struggling with will just pop into my head during one of my early morning yoga sessions.

All this talk of yogic and creative bliss brings us to the conundrum that surely an artist has to suffer for his or her art. There is some truth in this. When seeing a creative project through, from start to finish, there usually are numerous challenges along the way. To express yourself creatively takes courage, stamina, and a huge amount of self-belief. The moments of yogic bliss we experience might be fleeting; however, they sustain us when the going gets tough, and we have to navigate the inevitable obstacles that are strewn upon our path in life.

Create a Better World with Yoga and Creativity!

Renowned yogi T. K. V. Desikachar wrote, "A further meaning of the word *yoga* is 'to attain what was previously unattainable.'"[6] If you are dissatisfied with the way your life is going or concerned about the state of the world, then yoga combined with creativity will help you to act with love and power to transform the world around you. This is a path of lifelong learning.

Often the creative impulse is born from a sense of dissatisfaction with the way things are. The creative mind is a rebellious mind. It asks questions, it challenges societal norms, and although this does not lead to an easy life, it does lead to a more interesting one. Creativity empowers us to envision that the world could be different, that things could be done in a better way. Perhaps you are concerned that if you get too blissed out with yoga you will lose your creative edge. I can understand this concern, although

---

6. T. K. V. Desikachar, *The Heart of Yoga* (Rochester, VT: Inner Traditions, 1995), 5.

personally, I have found the opposite to be true. During over forty years of yoga practice, I have never lost my sense of indignation at the injustice in the world, but rather than feeling small and disempowered by this realization, yoga gives me the clarity to see the small steps that I can take to make changes in my life and the world.

It works both ways, and I have found that my creative, questioning mind has also kept me safe within the yoga world. There are some schools of yoga that discourage thinking for yourself; there is an emphasis on unquestioning obedience, with power coming from the top downward, which creates the perfect conditions for abuse to occur. I have sometimes found myself in such yoga environments and have made myself unpopular through asking questions. Fortunately, a combination of creative curiosity on my part, trust in my own inner wisdom, and a strong dose of feminism thrown in has meant that I have been able to navigate these challenging environments and steer myself onto a path of yoga that is authentic and wholesome.

Yoga, in its purest form, is subversive. In a world where we are encouraged to always be busy, to overconsume, to constantly divert ourselves, yoga beckons us to stop, to slow down, to reflect, to be present to this moment in time. This is a radical way of being that leads us to question the wisdom of always doing. We reconnect with the rhythms of nature, which are also our own rhythms. This is a saner way of being in the world and leads us to live in a way that is more sustainable for the planet.

Chakra-Inspired Yoga Practices

Each of the chakra chapters of the book has its own yoga practice. The seven chakra-inspired yoga practices are designed to encapsulate the essence of the chakra and to stimulate your creativity. Incorporated into the yoga practices are the element, color, and mantra that are associated with the chakra. Each chakra yoga practice also has its own affirmation. The following are some of the primary concerns that influence the design of each chakra-inspired yoga practice:

Root Chakra: Grounding and building strong foundations

Sacral Chakra: Fluidity, getting your energy flowing

Solar Plexus Chakra: Strength and empowerment

Heart Chakra: Heart opening, creating a loving space to hold and heal emotions

Throat Chakra: Expression, finding your voice

Third Eye Chakra: Developing intuition and clear sightedness

Crown Chakra: Opening to the possibility of bliss and enlightenment

To give you an example of how a chakra-inspired yoga practice is constructed, let's take a look at the root chakra. The element associated with the root chakra is earth, so we choose yoga poses that are grounding, such as Mountain Pose (*Tadasana*), Tree Pose (*Vrksasana*), and standing poses such as Warrior Pose (*Virabhadrasana*), Chair Pose (*Utkatasana*), and Standing Forward Bend (*Uttanasana*). We also cultivate an awareness of the lower body, which is associated with this chakra, sensing a connection to the earth through the feet, or whichever part of the body is in contact with the ground. We can incorporate the chakra's seed mantra *Lam* into dynamic yoga sequences. Or during the practice, you might visualize a red flower. In the book's root chakra-inspired yoga practice we use these two affirmations: *The earth supports me*, and *The earth nourishes me*. When we come to move up to the second chakra, the element here is water, and so we would choose fluid, flowing yoga sequences, for example.

Even if you are fairly new to yoga, you will find the yoga practices in the book easy to follow and accessible. All the practices are short enough to be able to fit into a busy day. If you are an experienced yogi, try out the practices in the book, and then use them as a jumping off point for creating your own chakra-inspired yoga practices.

CHAPTER 2

The Creative Power
of the Chakras

In Hindu literature the story that has been woven around the chakras is an epic one, involving a god and a goddess and a lovers' quest to be reunited. The goddess in question is Shakti, and she is the universal cosmic energy and the source of all creation. The god is Shiva, and he is pure consciousness. He is only whole and complete when she, Shakti, breathes life into him. Shiva without his Shakti is likened to a corpse. Shakti manifests within each human being as a snake that is coiled up at the base of the spine, called Kundalini. When awakened, Kundalini is the explosive creative potential, our spark of genius, that is contained within each one of us. She is said to be stronger than a million suns, and she lies latent, asleep, until she is awoken by the strong desire to be blissfully reunited with her lover, Shiva, who resides at the crown chakra.

Shakti is the cosmic creative energy that breathes life into matter and powers up the universe. So the next time you feel creatively blocked, evoke the power of Shakti to inspire and empower your creative journey. Shakti is thought to manifest in the form of Kundalini on the one hand and life force (*prana*) on the other. Kundalini is the fundamental potency behind all creativity. When Kundalini is awakened, she travels up the spine, piercing each of the chakras on her journey to be reunited with her lover, Shiva, who resides at the thousand-petaled lotus at the crown chakra. When we work with the chakras, we are learning to align ourselves with Shakti's primordial energy, which is the dynamic, feminine, creative principle of existence. So, by working with the power behind the chakras, you are harnessing the creative power of the universe and turbo-charging your creativity!

Tune In to Infinite Creative Energy with the Chakras

It was working with the chakras that first made me realize the amazing creative potential of yoga both on and off the mat. The chakras are a real treasure trove of inspiration for our creativity, encompassing colors, mandalas, sounds, gemstone, gods and goddesses, planets, and more. I found that my own home yoga practice and my teaching really blossomed and became so much more creative once I had begun to integrate the chakras into my practice. I'm certain that this flowering of creativity arose from working with the chakras and laid the foundations for developing my seasonal and zodiac-inspired approaches to yoga, and subsequently writing and publishing *Yoga Through the Year* and *Yoga by the Stars*.

In many ways the creative person has a head start when beginning to work with the chakras, precisely because she is used to working with that which cannot be seen and imagining it into existence. In the process of creation, the creative person works with both seen and unseen forces. The artist's masterpiece begins with a germ of an idea, a seed that is planted in the artist's mind that only she or he can see and which is invisible to others. The process by which the seed of an idea germinates, sends up green shoots, and eventually blossoms is a mysterious one. Imagination, creative vision, and limitless energy are required to see an idea through to fruition. We can use our yoga practice, in particular working with the chakras, to sharpen our creative vision, improve our imagination, and tune in to an infinite source of creative energy.

My love for the chakras was not a case of love at first sight; instead it was something that grew and blossomed over several years. Initially, my understanding of the chakras was mostly a cerebral one that I had acquired from reading learned books on the subject, combined with what I'd learned about the concept of the chakras when I was training to teach yoga. So although I understood the concept of the chakras on an intellectual level, they were mostly an abstract concept to me, and not one that I could relate to my own experience of yoga on or off the mat. However, gradually my understanding of the chakras changed from an abstract, intellectual idea to a living, embodied, creative reality.

So what was it that made the chakra system come to life for me? I love reading yoga books, and I came across a beautifully illustrated book on the subject. The visual images stimulated my imagination, and I began to be able to visualize the beauty and the creative potential of the chakra system. I also started introducing chakra meditations and visualizations into my own home yoga practice and into my teaching too. The old maxim of "An ounce of practice is worth a ton of theory" proved true here. However, I still think there is great value in studying the theory behind the chakra system through books, videos, or with a teacher, as this will provide a solid foundation for more creative practical explorations. Often in life we understand things on an intellectual level, and then over time that learning becomes integrated into our lives through practical lived experience.

I experienced another breakthrough regarding my understanding of the chakras when I was working on the Gemini chapter of my book *Yoga by the Stars*. Gemini is ruled by Mercury, the winged messenger of the gods, who carries a caduceus, which is a magic wand, entwined by two snakes and topped by a pair of wings. The caduceus is an ancient healing symbol and is still an international symbol for both the medical profession and homeopaths. Barbara Walker writes, "Hindu symbolism equated the caduceus with the central spirit of the human body, the spinal column, with the two mystic serpents twined around it … *ida-nadi* to the left, *pingala-nadi* to the right."[7]

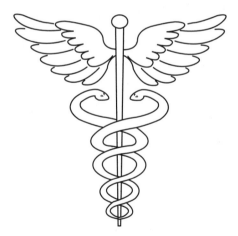

The Caduceus

7. Barbara G. Walker, *The Woman's Encyclopedia of Myths and Secrets* (New York: HarperCollins, 1983), 131.

It was meditating upon the symbol of the caduceus when I was devising a Gemini yoga practice, which opened my heart to the embodied nature of the chakras, transporting me from an intellectual understanding of the chakra system to a blissful lived experience of them.

In case you're not familiar with the esoteric anatomy envisaged by the ancient yogis, I'll outline it here. It centered around three primary channels (*nadis*) that were conduits of the life force (*prana*), with the central channel (*sushumna*), running through the center of the spine, and on either side the cooling moon channel (*ida-nadi*) and the heating sun channel (*pingala-nadi*), with self-realization being achieved once the serpent energy (*Kundalini*) had ascended from the base chakra, through the *sushumna*, to the chakra at the crown of the head.[8]

Of course, I was familiar with all the above, but it only really came alive for me in a tangible way after meditating upon the caduceus. It was during that spine-tingling meditation that the symbol of the caduceus morphed, in my mind's eye, into the Tree of Life, and it felt like my spine had become the center of that tree, flanked by the sun and moon on either side. From here the wings found at the tip of the caduceus wand effortlessly metamorphosized into higher consciousness, *samadhi*, which I experienced as a state of bliss, or self-realization.

The Poetic Symbolism of the Chakras

The chakra system has a poetic symbolism that we can draw upon to inspire our yoga practice and our creativity. The chakras map out a poetic, symbolic map of our inner solar system, helping us locate the constellations of our own subtle energy system. No one can define exactly what the chakras are or where they are located, so each time you work with the chakras, you are an explorer of inner space.

Each time we meditate upon the chakras and visualize them manifesting within our body, we are creating an interface between the seen material world and the unseen world of subtle energy and spirit. Each time that we tune in to and imagine a chakra as a colored light, a lotus flower, a sacred sound, or an archetype, we are balancing our sun and moon energies, bringing heaven down to earth and raising earth up to heaven, and so uniting the visible world of matter with the invisible world of spirit.

There are seven main chakras along the midline of the body. The chakras were envisioned by the Tantric yogis as spinning vortices of psychospiritual energy that formed

---

8. Georg Feuerstein, *Encyclopedic Dictionary of Yoga* (New York: Paragon House, 1990), 143, 228, 259, and 354.

part of a network of subtle energy found within the human body. The yogis conceived of the chakras as wheels that connected the world of spirit and matter and provided an interface between the heavenly and earthly realms. The Tantric yogis intuited the location of the chakras in the body and through the power of their imagination created an anatomical map of the body's subtle energy system and uncovered its relationship to both the spiritual and material domains. This anatomical description of the subtle energy system is symbolic and poetic and serves to help the yogi climb the steps to enlightenment, by increasing awareness and bringing about a transformation that leads to a state of unsurpassed bliss (*ananda*).

This poetic model of the chakras, as opposed to a literal one, gives us the freedom to intuit where the chakras are in the body and to allow our imagination to roam free. We find that in the silent stillness of meditation, a door opens, leading into the subconscious and universal conscious. In this deeply relaxed, awakened yogic state we gain access to the body's subtle energy centers (chakras) which in turn are a doorway to the soul.

The chakras are wheels or vortices of energy that store the universal life force (prana). The actual spelling of chakra is *cakra*, but this spelling is not commonly used. *Cakra* ("wheel") is derived from the verbal root *car* ("to move"). There are seven main chakras located along the midline of the body between the base of the spinal column and the crown of the head. Some sources wrongly interpret the chakras as nerve plexuses; however, the scriptural testimony of Tantric yogic authorities contradicts this literal interpretation.[9] The chakras are "centers of psychospiritual energy that don't precisely correspond to any tangible physical structure."[10] The chakras are imagined into being by the Tantric yogi as an aid to meditation. The beauty of this interpretation means that each one of us can visualize and create a chakra system that is guided by yogic principles but ultimately uniquely our own, which is in itself a profoundly creative act.

On the next page is a chart showing the main creative concern of the chakras.

---

9. Feuerstein, *Encyclopedic Dictionary of Yoga*, 72–73.

10. Joan Budilovsky and Eve Adamson, *The Complete Idiot's Guide to Yoga* (Indianapolis, IN: Alpha Books 2001), 231.

Creative Concerns of the Chakras						
Chakra	*Meaning*	*Location*	*Associated Color*	*Main Creative Concern of Chakra*	*Bija Mantra*	*Associated Element*
Root Chakra (*Muladhara*)	Root or support	Base of the spine	Red	Developing a stable base to create from.	*Lam*	Earth
Sacral Chakra (*Svadhisthana*)	One's own abode, sweetness	Lower abdomen	Orange	Riding the ebb and flow of creativity. Seeking and giving pleasure through your work.	*Vam*	Water
Solar Plexus Chakra (*Manipura*)	Lustrous gem	Upper abdomen	Yellow	Firing up your creativity with confidence and empowerment.	*Ram*	Fire
Heart Chakra (*Anahata*)	Wheel of the unstruck sound	At the heart	Pink, green	Creating with love and compassion for self and others.	*Yam*	Air
Communication Chakra (*Vishuddha*)	Pure wheel	The throat	Blue	Giving voice to your creations and communicating your vision.	*Ham*	Ether
Third Eye Chakra (*Ajna*)	Command wheel	Between the brows	Indigo	Seeing intuitively with the inner eye and developing imagination.	*Am* or *Om*	Light
Crown Chakra (*Sahasrara*)	Thousand-spoked wheel	The space just above the crown of the head	Violet, gold, white	Creating from a state of pure bliss. Drawing from an infinite source of inspiration.	*Om*	Consciousness

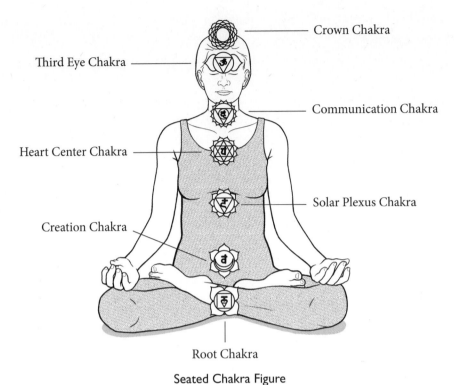

Crown Chakra

Third Eye Chakra

Communication Chakra

Heart Center Chakra

Solar Plexus Chakra

Creation Chakra

Root Chakra

Seated Chakra Figure

Developing Awareness of the Chakras

Imagine that you'd never tasted chocolate before. I could try describing it to you in words, but the best way for you to experience chocolate would be for you to taste it. Likewise, the best way for you to understand the chakras is through direct experience, and the following three meditations will give you a taste of locating the chakras in your body.

EXERCISE

Chakra Awareness Meditation

This meditation forms a basis for all the other chakra meditations in the book. It is a foundational practice that will enable you to locate within your body the psychoenergetic field of each of the seven chakras. It is a simple, enjoyable way of connecting with and tuning in to the seven main chakras. It is important to become familiar with this meditation before you go on to work with the other chakra meditations, as all the following chakra meditations begin with this simple step of tuning in to each of the seven chakras, which you learn to do in this meditation.

The Chakra Awareness Meditation works well as a standalone practice, can be used at the beginning or end of a yoga session, and can be used to begin or conclude any of the yoga practices in this book. The meditation is grounding and centering. It has a purifying effect on the chakras, shifting stuck, stagnant energy, clearing blocked subtle energy channels, and helping energy flow freely.

I'd like to encourage you to approach this meditation with curiosity and to let go of the notion that there is a correct way to do it. The ancient yogis developed the chakra model as an aid to meditation. It's important to remember when you are doing this meditation that the chakras are a poetic, symbolic representation of wheels of energy, rather than exact physical locations that can be pinpointed within the body. Allow your inner wisdom and intuition to guide you to the exact location of each chakra within your body. After a while you will easily be able to zoom into and locate each of the chakras every time you meditate on them.

Allow 10 minutes.

In this meditation we take our awareness from the root chakra, at the base of the spine, up the length of the spine to the crown chakra at the top of the head. We sequentially bring our awareness to, and feel into, the part of the body where each chakra is located.

To begin, find yourself a comfortable position: either an erect sitting position or lying on the floor in Relaxation Pose (*Savasana*). Whichever position you choose, take a minute to ground yourself. Be aware of where your body is in contact with the floor or your support. Relax into the support of the earth beneath you.

In this meditation you are going to direct the spotlight of your awareness along the midline of the body, tuning in to each of the seven chakras in turn. As you tune in to the physical location associated with the chakra, be aware of any physical sensations, thoughts, feelings, or visual images that arise.

1. Bring your awareness to the root chakra. This chakra is associated with the lower body. Be aware of the pelvis, the legs, and the feet. Now tune in to the base of the spine, the anus, the pelvic floor, and the sexual organs, noticing any sensations that are present here. The root chakra is your foundation, rooting you and giving you support. Intuitively

feel into and locate the center of this spinning circle of psychospiritual energy, and as you do so, be aware of any physical sensations, thoughts, feelings, or visual images that arise.

2. Now bring your awareness to the sacral chakra. Be aware of the lower abdomen, the sacrum, and the parts of your body that you associate with fertility and sexual pleasure. Intuitively feel into the center of the sacral chakra's circle, being aware of any physical sensations, thoughts, feelings, or visual images that arise.

3. Bring your awareness to the solar plexus chakra, which is your center of personal power. Tune in to the upper abdomen, particularly the area between the navel and the base of the breastbone, along the midline of the body. Intuitively feel into the center of the circle of energy that is your solar plexus chakra, being aware of any physical sensations, thoughts, feelings, or visual images that arise.

4. Bring your awareness to the heart chakra, which is the center of your loving and compassionate heart. Tune in to the area around the heart, lungs, ribcage, and thoracic spine. Intuitively feel into the center of the circle of your heart chakra, being aware of any physical sensations, thoughts, feelings, or visual images that arise.

5. Bring your awareness to the communication chakra, which is the center of your creative expression in the world. Feel into the area around your neck, throat, mouth, and both ears. Intuitively feel into the center of the circle that is your communication chakra, and be aware of any physical sensations, thoughts, feelings, or visual images that arise.

6. Bring your awareness to the third eye chakra, which is the center of clear-sightedness, clairvoyance, intuition, and imagination. Tune in to the area between the brows, the eyes, and behind the eyes. Intuitively feel into the center of the circle of energy that is your third eye chakra, and be aware of any physical sensations, thoughts, feelings, or visual images that arise.

7. Bring your awareness to the crown chakra, which is the center for self-realization and transcendence. Tune in to the space just above the crown of the head. Intuitively feel into the center of the circle of energy

that is your crown chakra, being aware of any physical sensations, thoughts, feelings, or visual images that arise.

Then repeat the steps in reverse order, from 7 back to 1. Observe how you are feeling having completed the meditation. Ground yourself by noticing the sensations associated with where your body is in contact with the floor or your support.

You can conclude the meditation with the Chakra-Closing Lotus Visualization that follows.

EXERCISE

Chakra-Closing Lotus Visualization

All the chakra meditations in this book can be concluded with the Chakra-Closing Lotus Visualization. The picturing of the chakras closing that we use in this visualization ensures that we are not too open after working with the chakras and that we have the necessary psychic protection in place to function well in our everyday life.

If you are lying, come back to sitting. Bring your hands together in the Prayer Position (*Namaste*) at the heart center. Then from the Prayer Position make your hands and fingers into the shape of a fully open lotus flower (*Padma Mudra*). Then gently curl the fingers so the hands look like a flower closing back to bud. As you do this, picture all your seven chakras closing back to bud too. Repeat three times, inhaling as your hand flower opens and exhaling as it closes back to bud.

EXERCISE

Chakra Colored Light Visualization

In this visualization we focus our awareness on each chakra in turn and visualize a colored light at the chakra. We picture the light being the color that is traditionally associated with each chakra. Here is a reminder of the colors associated with the chakras:

Root Chakra: Red

Sacral Chakra: Orange

Solar Plexus Chakra: Yellow

Heart Chakra: Pink or green

Communication Chakra: Blue

Third Eye Chakra: Indigo

Crown Chakra: Violet, gold, or white

This visualization will help you develop your ability to visualize and sense the chakras. It is uplifting, is gently energizing, encourages the free flow of subtle energy (prana), and induces a sense of well-being.

The Chakra Colored Light Visualization can be used as a standalone practice, or it can be used at the end of a yoga session, and it can be used to conclude any of the yoga practices in this book.

To begin, find yourself a comfortable position: either an erect sitting position or lying on the floor in Relaxation Pose (*Savasana*). Whichever position you choose, take a minute to ground yourself. Be aware of where your body is in contact with the floor or your support. Relax into the support of the earth beneath you.

In this meditation you are going to take your awareness along the midline of the body, tuning in to each of the seven chakras in turn and visualizing a colored light radiating at each chakra. As you tune in to the chakra, be aware of any physical sensations, thoughts, feelings, or visual images that arise.

The chakras are said to be located within the subtle energy channel, called the *sushumna*, that runs along the center of the spinal column. So before you start, take a moment to take your awareness along the length of the *sushumna*, from the base of the spine up through the center of the spine, to the crown of the head, and then from the crown of the head back down along the center of the spine, to the base of the spine.

1. Bring your awareness to the root chakra, tuning in to the area around the base of the spine, the anus, the pelvic floor, and the sexual organs. As you tune in to the area, simultaneously visualize a glowing red light where you sense the location of the root chakra is situated, being aware of any physical sensations, thoughts, feelings, or visual images that arise as you do this.

2. Now bring your awareness to the sacral chakra along the midline, in the lower abdomen, and visualize an orange light here, being aware of any physical sensations, thoughts, feelings, or visual images that arise.

3. Bring your awareness to the solar plexus chakra, tuning in to the area of the spine between the navel and the base of the breastbone, visualizing a yellow light shining here, being aware of any physical sensations, thoughts, feelings, or visual images that arise.

4. Bring your awareness to the heart chakra and visualize either a green or pink light glowing here, being aware of any physical sensations, thoughts, feelings, or visual images that arise.

5. Bring your awareness to the communication chakra, feeling into the area around your neck, throat, mouth, and both ears, picturing a blue light here, being aware of any physical sensations, thoughts, feelings, or visual images that arise.

6. Bring your awareness to the third eye chakra, tuning in to the area between the brows, visualizing an indigo light here, being aware of any physical sensations, thoughts, feelings, or visual images that arise.

7. Bring your awareness to the crown chakra, tuning in to the space just above the crown of the head, picturing a violet, white, or gold light here, being aware of any physical sensations, thoughts, feelings, or visual images that arise.

Then imagine that rays of golden sunlight are shining down from above and radiating around your entire body. Then repeat the steps above, in reverse order, from 7 back to 1. Observe how you are feeling having completed the meditation. Ground yourself by noticing the sensations associated with where your body is in contact with the floor or your support.

You can conclude the meditation with the Chakra-Closing Lotus Visualization (see page 26).

The Chakras and Sacred Sound

It can be rewarding to work with the seed (*bija*) mantras associated with each chakra. They are so simple … and you don't even need to have a tuneful voice to join in! I've integrated the seed mantras into several of the chakra-inspired yoga practices and meditations in this book. They combine well with simple yoga movements and give a meditative focus to the practice.

Below is a reminder of the seed mantras and their related chakras.

Root Chakra: *Lam* (pronounced *lum*)

Sacral Chakra: *Vam* (pronounced *vum*)

Solar Plexus Chakra: *Ram* (pronounced *rum*)

Heart Chakra: *Yam* (pronounced *yum*)

Communication Chakra: *Ham* (pronounced *hum*)

Third Eye Chakra: *Am* (pronounced *um*)

Crown Chakra: *Om* (pronounced *a-u-m*)

To get a feel for working with them, try the following Chakra Seed-Mantra Meditation.

EXERCISE
Chakra Seed-Mantra Meditation

This meditation gives a simple, enjoyable way of connecting with the seven main chakras. It works well at the end of a yoga session, and it could be used to conclude any of the chakra yoga practices in this book. The meditation helps shift stuck, stagnant energy, clearing blocked subtle energy channels and allowing energy to flow more freely.

Allow 10 minutes.

In this meditation we take our awareness from the root chakra at the base of the spine up to the crown chakra at the top of the head. We sequentially bring our awareness to, and feel into, the part of the body where the chakra is located, and then we repeat three times the *bija* mantra associated with that chakra.

If meditating lying down, we use the seed mantras silently. This is exquisitely relaxing as well as gently energizing. If done sitting, the seed mantras can be vocalized, repeated silently internally, or a combination of both. I like to vocalize the mantras from the root chakra up to the crown of the head and then repeat the mantras silently on the journey down from crown of head back to the root chakra at the base of the spine.

To begin, find yourself a comfortable position: either an erect sitting position or lying on the floor in Relaxation Pose (*Savasana*).

1. Bring your awareness to the base of the spine. Feel into this area and notice any sensations that are present. On the exhale, repeat the mantra *Lam* (pronounced *lum*) three times, either silently or out loud.

2. Bring your awareness to the lower abdomen. Feel into this area and notice any sensations that are present. Repeat the mantra *Vam* (pronounced *vum*) three times, either silently or out loud.

3. Bring your awareness to the upper abdomen. Feel into this area and notice any sensations that are present. Repeat the mantra *Ram* (pronounced *rum*) three times, either silently or out loud.

4. Bring your awareness to the heart center. Feel into this area and notice any sensations that are present. Repeat the mantra *Yam* (pronounced *yum*) three times, either silently or out loud.

5. Bring your awareness to the throat. Feel into this area and notice any sensations that are present. Repeat the mantra *Ham* (pronounced *hum*) three times, either silently or out loud.

6. Bring your awareness to between the brows. Feel into this area and notice any sensations that are present. Repeat the mantra *Am* (pronounced *um*) three times, either silently or out loud.

7. Bring your awareness to the space just above the crown of the head. Feel into this area and notice any sensations that are present. Repeat the mantra *Om* (pronounced *aum*), three times, either silently or out loud.

Then repeat the steps in reverse order, from 7 back to 1. Observe how you are feeling having completed the meditation. Ground yourself by noticing the sensations associated with where your body is in contact with the floor or your support.

You can conclude the meditation with the Chakra-Closing Lotus Visualization (see page 26).

The Mantras Om and Ma: The Mother Mantras

Each day, I finish my own yoga practice with several repetitions of the mantra *Om*, followed by several repetitions of the mantra *Ma*. Both mantras are nurturing and nourishing and provide us with a simple, enjoyable way of working with the chakras.

The mantras are an excellent way of stilling the mind and uplifting the spirit. They can be vocalized or silently repeated.

Om is a deeply feminine mantra, referred to in the Upanishads as "the supreme syllable, the mother of all sound." Its meaning is something like "pregnant belly," and the mantra is imbued with such creative power that it was uttered by the Great Goddess as a spell to bring the world into being.[11]

In Indo-European languages *Ma* is universally known as the basic mother word. *Ma* was often defined in the Far East as the "spark of life" or intelligence.[12] Repetition of the mantra *Ma* induces a sense of being protected, supported, sustained, and connected to the umbilical cord of life.

PRACTICE

Mantra *Om*

Repetition of the manta *Om* takes us on a journey from the lower to the higher chakras. The vibrations from the mantra are healing and shift stuck energy. The mantra is energizing and uplifting, the breathing is deepened, and concentration and focus are improved. The muscles around the face, neck, and throat are exercised. The mantra gives our creative process a boost, as we become accustomed to expressing ourselves whilst maintaining a meditative frame of mind.

Allow 10 minutes.

Find yourself a comfortable, erect seated position. If you have not practiced this mantra before, then begin with step 1. However, if you are familiar with the mantra, go straight to step 2.

1. The mantra *Om* is made up of three sounds, a-u-m (*ah-ooh-mm*). To familiarize yourself with the sounds, begin by sounding each sound separately.

    Inhale. On the exhale make the *ah* sound, dropping your awareness to the pelvic basin and feeling the vibration of the sound there. As you complete the sound, allow a slight, silent pause, and then relax as the breath fills your lungs. Repeat 3 times.

11. Barbara G. Walker, *The Woman's Dictionary of Symbols and Sacred Objects* (New York: HarperCollins, 1988), 99.

12. Walker, *The Woman's Encyclopedia of Myths and Secrets*, 560.

Then inhale. On the exhale make the *ooh* sound, bringing your awareness to the chest cavity and experiencing the vibration of the sound there. As you complete the sound, allow a slight, silent pause, and then relax as the breath fills your lungs. Repeat 3 times.

Then inhale. On the exhale make the *mm* sound, prolonging the sound and feeling the vibration of the sound in the skull. As you complete the sound, allow a slight, silent pause, and then relax as the breath fills your lungs. Repeat 3 times.

Now you are ready to go on to step 2 and put these three sounds together to make the *Om* sound (*ah-ooh-mm*).

2. Inhale, on the exhale make the *Om* sound (*ah-ooh-mm*). As you make the sound, your awareness travels up the body from the pelvic basin, through the chest cavity, to the skull. *Ah*, pelvic basin. *Ooh*, chest cavity. *Mm*, skull. As you complete the *Om* sound, allow a slight, silent pause, and then relax as the breath fills your lungs.

Repeat 3 or more times. If you are finishing your practice here, just sit quietly for a few breaths, noticing what effect the practice has had on you. Or follow this practice with a few repetitions of the mantra *Ma*, which follows.

PRACTICE
Mantra *Ma*

I like to follow repetitions of the mantra *Om* with several repetitions of the mantra *Ma*. It is a wonderfully grounding mantra that gently guides our awareness down from the head and into the lower body. It's also a nurturing, nourishing way to conclude any yoga session.

Allow 3 to 5 minutes. Find yourself a comfortable, erect seated position.

Inhale, and on the exhale make the *Ma* sound, dividing it into two syllables, *mm* and *ah*. On the *mm* sound, feel the vibration of the sound in the skull. On a prolonged *ah* sound, drop your awareness to the pelvic basin, and feel the vibration of the sound there.

Repeat 3 or more times. Then sit quietly for a few breaths, enjoying the silence and noticing what effect the practice has had on you.

CHAPTER 3

Mindful Walking to Unlock Your Creative Potential

When I am writing a book or involved in any other creative endeavor, walking is one of my greatest allies. My main reason for walking is that I love walking. I find that walking is an act of self-kindness, and it's a huge part of my creative process. Most days I walk about three miles in the fresh air, but I also intersperse my writing sessions with periods of indoor walking meditation, and I find this is a great way to stay fresh and keep my ideas flowing while I write.

In this section I will share with you some ways of using walking, both formally and informally, to boost your creative powers. In each of the chakra chapters you will find a chakra-inspired walking meditation:

Root Chakra: Awareness of the feet and contact with the earth when walking. Walk as if your feet are kissing the earth.

Sacral Chakra: Walking with breath awareness and seeking out what you find pleasurable.

Solar Plexus Chakra: Solar-powered walking meditation, with sun visualization, to build confidence and to promote a sunny attitude.

Heart Chakra: Compassionate walking meditation, extending love and compassion to yourself and others as you walk.

Communication Chakra: Mindfulness of sound walking meditation.

Third Eye Chakra: Slow, mindful walking, appreciating the beauty around you and looking with fresh eyes.

Crown Chakra: Blissful walking meditation, honing your capacity to find joy in a million small, everyday experiences.

Walking as a Creative Superpower!

As a writer, I spend many hours of each day in front of a screen, I counterbalance the mental and physical stress that this causes by interspersing periods of writing with periods of walking meditation, and this has the added benefit of keeping me fit and healthy while I work on a book, and it also improves my writing, as following a period of walking meditation, I return to my desk refreshed and buzzing with ideas.

Walking can boost your creativity and be an important aspect of self-care during the creative process. For centuries writers, artists, musicians, mathematicians, and scientists have instinctively known what scientific research now confirms: that walking helps with problem-solving and generating creative solutions. In his book *In Praise of Walking*, Professor Shane O'Mara writes, "If we want to encourage freer forms of creative cognition, we need to get people up from their desks, away from their screens, and get them moving." We can, he says, create "a more creative state … by being in motion."[13]

The philosopher Friedrich Nietzsche even said, "Only thoughts *won by walking* are valuable."[14] When we walk, the earth supports us and heaven inspires us. Many writers find that they get their best ideas when out walking and write better after a period of walking. Walking boosts your brain power because it increases blood flow to the brain, which in turn has cognitive benefits. This explains why many of us find that we can solve a problem and generate creative solutions on a walk.

For Virginia Woolf walking and writing were inseparable. She made up her books as she walked along. Poet William Wordsworth composed "Lines Written a Few Miles above Tintern Abbey" while walking. Since antiquity, it has been recognized that a good

---

13. Shane O'Mara, *In Praise of Walking* (London: Penguin Random House, 2019), 157.

14. Friedrich Nietzsche, *Twilight of the Idols and the Antichrist*, trans. Thomas Common (Mineola, NY: Dover, 2004), 7.

walk is an excellent way to think problems through. "The school of peripatetic philosophy in ancient Greece was famous for conducting its teaching largely on foot, and the root of its name means 'walking up and down,'" shares O'Mara.[15]

From a young age I learned that walking was a wonderful way to relieve stress. During my childhood and adolescence, my late father had severe mental health problems, which meant his behavior was irrational, unpredictable, and frightening; consequently, I always felt safer outside of the house rather than inside. Walking outside became a place of refuge for me. I was fortunate that beginning when I was eight years old, we lived opposite three square miles of parkland. During my childhood, I got to know every inch of that park by heart. Sometimes with friends, sometimes on my own, I climbed trees, I slid down mudbanks, I picked bluebells, I kicked through autumn leaves, and I was delighted when snow fell. Although I was a townie, the park allowed me to connect with nature and was somewhere that I felt safe and at home.

Nowadays, I find that walking clears my head, helps me generate ideas, and frees up my imagination. I walk to stay healthy, relieve stress, process the events of daily life, ponder themes I am writing about, and be out in the fresh air and to connect with nature. Walking is a natural mood booster. Virginia Woolf wrote in her diaries how she was able to walk herself calm and serene again.[16] In an article for *Women & Home,* Faye Smith states that "when researchers asked people with depression to walk for 30 minutes three times a week for 16 weeks, they found it had similar mood-boosting effects to antidepressant medication."[17] Walking is medicine! Walking can improve your sleep and lower your risk of experiencing diabetes, high blood pressure, heart disease, strokes, and obesity. Walking supports heart and lung health through cardiovascular exercise, and "it strengthens the primary muscles of your lower limbs and aids in maintaining healthy bone density."[18]

A large part of creative thinking is the ability to create something new by combining ideas in a surprising and novel way. The creative person perceives the world in new

---

15. O'Mara, *In Praise of Walking,* 145.

16. Alexandra Harris, "Sussex," *A Walk of One's Own: Virginia Woolf on Foot*, episode 4, BBC Radio, September 1, 2015, radio broadcast, 13:51, https://www.bbc.co.uk/sounds/play/b067wnnd.

17. Faye M. Smith, "Benefits of Walking: 7 Reasons Why It's Extremely Good for Your Health," *Woman & Home*, October 23, 2020, https://www.womanandhome.com/health-and-well-being/health-benefits-of-walking-385528/.

18. Smith, "Benefits of Walking."

ways, finds hidden patterns, and makes connections between seemingly unrelated phenomena. One of the ways that walking boosts our creativity is that while our bodies are involved in the rhythmic, hypnotic action of putting one foot in front of the other, our minds are free to roam. Over the duration of a walk, our mind might flit from the past to the future, and like a butterfly it will land on one subject, perhaps the beauty of a flower, or notice clouds rushing across a blue sky, and then it will flit onto another subject, such as the state of the world today or what we are going to eat for dinner.

The Mindful Approach to Creative Walking

The simplest way of taking advantage of the amazing creative potential and health benefits of walking is just to make some time each day to get outside in the fresh air and walk. When I'm outside I like to walk at a brisk pace, although not so fast that I am unable to take in the world around me. Especially after long periods of being at my desk writing, it's great to be outside, to feast my eyes on the beauty of the changing seasons, to feel a cool breeze or warm sunshine on my face, to let my imagination run wild as I read meaning into the faces of passing strangers.

Some people like to count their steps with a pedometer. Personally, I prefer to approach walking in the same way that I approach a yoga session: gently monitoring and observing my bodily sensations and the thoughts and feelings that are passing through my mind.

So we've established that walking is a phenomenal way to boost creativity and that it also improves our health and sense of well-being. However, I would like to encourage you to walk for the pure joy of walking rather than walking to achieve a specific outcome. Keep this in mind as you read the following descriptions outlining the different approaches to creative walking used in this book.

The following are two foundational walking meditations. They will give you an experience of using walking meditation to boost your creativity and will help you establish an inspiring, mindful walking habit. It would be a good idea to familiarize yourself with these two meditations before going on to try the chakra-inspired walking meditations contained within each of the chakra chapters of this book.

EXERCISE

Formal Walking Meditation

When I am in the middle of writing a book, I use this formal walking meditation every day, and sometimes a few times during the day. I usually follow the walking meditation with a writing meditation. I find it a great way of getting my ideas flowing, generating ideas, and finding creative solutions to problems. It also has the added benefit of keeping me fit while I'm writing (so much so, that I actually lost a few pounds of weight while writing this book!).

A formal walking meditation involves walking meditatively on a specific circuit for a specified amount of time. Your walking circuit could be inside or outside and might involve walking from one side of a room to the other and back again or walking in a circle. Choose somewhere you feel safe and will not be disturbed, such as a room in your house, a hallway, your garden, a local park, an unused room at your gym, or a corridor at work. I'm fortunate to have the house to myself during the day, so my walking circuit runs across the length of my kitchen, through my writing room, and across my sitting room, and then I retrace my steps back to the kitchen again.

It's a good idea to set a timer and commit to walking for a specific amount of time. Ten minutes is ideal, but you can do more if you wish.

Start the meditation by becoming aware of how it feels to walk, noticing the contact between your feet and the ground beneath you, and any sensations you feel in the feet. Keep a background awareness of how your whole body feels as you walk. Maintain a gentle awareness of the natural flow of your breath. Take enjoyment from the act of walking.

You can choose to walk with a specific meditative focus, or you can walk without a specific focus. Here's some guidance on that:

Walking with Focus

If you have a specific creative dilemma that you are hoping to solve, then you can focus on this as you walk. Notice any ideas that come into your head in response to the chosen theme. Feel free to explore these ideas and see where they lead you. Be gently vigilant, and if you notice your attention getting hijacked by everyday preoccupations, concerns, and worries, just gently but firmly lead it back to the subject. Enjoy exploring any ideas that surface in response to your chosen theme.

Walking without a Focus

Alternatively, you can choose to walk and simply allow your mind to wander freely. Gently divide your attention between an awareness of how it feels to be walking, an awareness of your surroundings, and the thoughts and feelings that pass through your mind. Do not direct your attention to a particular focus; simply allow your mind to wander where it will. Watch and observe your mind as it flits from subject to subject, perhaps going over a problem, thinking about the future, or reliving events from the past. If you find yourself becoming carried away with the drama of your thoughts, shift your focus back to an awareness of how it feels to be walking, noticing the contact that your feet make with the earth with every step.

When your timer goes, at the end of your walking meditation, you might want to jot down any ideas, inspiration, or insights that came to you. Or, if you have time, follow this formal walking meditation with a writing meditation.

EXERCISE

Informal Walking Meditation

An informal walking meditation can be done either indoors or out, anytime you have to walk somewhere. It can be done in your house or office or when walking from your car to home or workplace. It can be done in the city, the country, a park, or a shopping mall. Do remember to stay safe and be aware of any hazards as you walk.

You begin the meditation by slightly slowing your walking down, but not so slow that you draw attention to yourself. Notice how it feels to be walking, especially the contact between your feet and the earth beneath you. Maintain a gentle awareness of your natural breathing as you walk. Take a sensual enjoyment in your surroundings, noticing the sights, sounds, and aromas.

You can choose to walk with a specific meditative focus, or you can walk without a specific focus. For guidance on this, see the instructions for the Formal Walking Meditation.

At the end of your walk, you might want to jot down any inspiration, ideas, or insights that surfaced during your meditation. Or if you have time, follow this informal walking meditation with a writing meditation.

* * *

In the chakra chapters you'll find a chakra-inspired walking meditation for each of the chakras. Also, check out the resources list at the end of the book for some suggestions for excellent books on walking meditation.

CHAPTER 4

Write Your Way to Happiness and Healing

In the spring of 2020, I spent a lot of time walking, writing, and crying. In the early part of the year both my parents had died within a few weeks of each other. I experienced a tsunami of grief, and as a survivor of childhood abuse, my grieving process was complicated and messy. Later in this chapter I will describe how walking and writing meditation helped me deal with and emerge from the trauma. I want to share the methods I used to help in my recovery from trauma, because I know from my own experience that repressing traumatic memories creates a block to our creative expression. Conversely, when we work through the trauma, our creativity is freed to grow and blossom.

However, you do not need to have suffered from trauma to benefit from the type of writing meditation that I will share with you in this chapter. Journaling, a form of writing therapy, has enjoyed a huge resurgence of popularity recently. This is not surprising because therapeutic writing is a great way to boost your creativity and enhance your well-being, regardless of whether you are a painter, a musician, a sculptor, or a scientist. And if you are suffering from some sort of creative block, expressive forms of writing can shift the block and help you generate new ideas.

Studies show that therapeutic writing reduces stress, boosts your mood, reduces symptoms of depression, and helps manage anxiety, shares Courtney Ackerman of PositivePsychology.com. Studies suggest that writing therapy can strengthen the immune system, lower blood pressure, improve sleep, and generally promote good health. It also helps your creativity "flourish and expand," and the reason for this is "journaling requires the application of the analytical, rational left side of the brain; while your left hemisphere is occupied, your right hemisphere (the creative, touchy-feely side) is given the freedom to wander and play."[19]

When I'm working on a book, if I get stuck with a chapter, I find the best way to shift the block and to generate new ideas is to use a combination of walking meditation and writing meditation. Likewise, if I am facing a challenge in life and I am unsure which direction to take, I find that walking and writing meditations help me generate creative solutions, boost my problem-solving skills, and help me move forward with my life.

You can use all the writing meditations in this chapter on their own; however, I find they are most effective if you precede them with a walking meditation (go back to chapter 3 for all the amazing benefits of walking on creativity). My own recipe for getting creative juices flowing is ten minutes of walking meditation followed by fifteen minutes of writing meditation.

Next, I will describe two forms of writing meditation. In the first, Free-Flow Writing Meditation, you do not have a specific focus, while in the second, Writing Meditation with Focus, you do. Both meditations can be done as standalone practices, can follow a sitting or walking meditation, or can be done before or after your yoga practice. Both writing meditations are effective ways to get your ideas flowing and allow you to gain access to the wisdom of your subconscious mind. If your creativity is blocked, the meditations will fire up your imagination. If you have come to an impasse in your life, they will help you reorient and get you moving forward again. You will also find chakra-inspired writing meditation suggestions in each of the chakra chapters of the book.

Your meditative writing will be more fruitful if you can cultivate the following qualities and skills and bring these attitudes to the meditation process:

- Curiosity
- Patience

---

19. Courtney Ackerman, "83 Benefits of Journaling for Depression, Anxiety, and Stress," PositivePsychology .com, May 2, 2021, https://positivepsychology.com/benefits-of-journaling/.

- Self-acceptance
- Self-compassion
- A sense of humor
- Listening skills
- An open mind

Personally, I like the physicality of writing with pen and paper. However, it's fine to work digitally too. Either way, have your writing materials on hand.

EXERCISE

Free-Flow Writing Meditation

This form of writing meditation is sometimes known as automatic writing or flow of consciousness writing. It has a cathartic effect, clears the mind, and opens the way for new ideas to surface.

The object of this meditation is not to pen a polished piece of writing, but rather simply to observe and record thoughts and feelings as they arise. The writing does not have to be smart, clever, witty, or even interesting. All you are required to do is to listen, observe, and be present to whatever arises in your mind during the allocated meditation period, and your job is to simply get this down on paper.

Be reassured that whatever you write during the meditation is for your eyes only. No need to pay attention to handwriting, neatness, spelling, grammar, presentation, and so on. As long as your writing is legible and comprehensible to you, anything goes.

Find yourself a comfortable position. Before you start writing, bring your awareness to your body, and notice any bodily sensations that are arising. Be aware of where your body is in contact with the floor or the chair. Now, bring your awareness to the natural flow of your breath. During the meditation, maintain a background awareness of your body and your breath.

Then set your timer for 10 to 20 minutes … and … start writing. Keep your pen in contact with the paper at all times and keep writing until your timer goes.

Write down whatever comes into your head. Your aim is to capture the stream of thoughts and feelings as they flow through your mind. Let go of your inner editor! It doesn't matter how off the wall your thoughts are—just get them down!

Later, after the meditation has finished, you can read the writing and see if there are any nuggets of gold among the stones and grit. But for now, just keep that pen moving!

Be aware of the physical act of writing and how it feels to be someone sitting here writing. Relax any parts of your body that do not need to be engaged with the act of writing. If you find that you are tensing up, slow your writing down, consciously relax, and reconnect with the flow of your breath. At the same time, keep writing! A relaxed attitude will help you access your subconscious mind, and it is here that we uncover our gold.

However, it's no problem if you find it impossible to relax—just keep on writing anyway. Part of your meditation can be to write and at the same time maintain a gentle awareness of how it feels to be tense, noticing sensations as they arise in your body. If you can't let it go, then just let it be.

Once your timer goes, put your pen down. Notice how your body feels, how you are feeling in yourself, and the natural flow of your breath. Be aware of where your body is in contact with the floor or your chair. And when you are ready, carry on with your day.

EXERCISE

Writing Meditation with Focus

Generally, I do ten minutes of Formal Walking Meditation (see page 37) before I do the Writing Meditation with Focus. I find the walking really frees up my mind and gets my creative juices flowing. However, it's fine to do this writing meditation as a standalone practice too.

Whereas in the previous meditation you allowed the mind to roam freely, in this meditation you choose a subject to focus on and keep bringing the mind back to that focus when it inevitably wanders off. So, for example, if I were designing a yoga practice for the root chakra, I might choose to do a writing meditation focusing on the theme of earth, which is the root chakra's element. In the meditation I would let my mind wander wherever it wanted as long as it was roughly related to the theme of earth. If my mind wandered off onto planning what I would have for lunch or noticing that the floor needed sweeping, then I would gently bring it back to the topic of earth. This is a meditative technique called "notice and return." You notice your mind has wandered and you gently return it to the chosen point of focus.

The Writing Meditation with Focus is exceptionally good training for developing the concentration and focus that you need to complete any creative project. Also, I'm sure you'll be bedazzled at the amazing power of the subconscious mind to come up with unexpected and original associations related to the theme you are focusing on. I find when doing this meditation that I frequently have "aha!" lightbulb moments, when a surprising, brilliant idea pops into my mind, as if plucked from thin air!

As with the previous meditation, be reassured that whatever you write down during this meditation is for your eyes only. No need to pay attention to handwriting, neatness, spelling, grammar, presentation, and so on. As long as your writing is legible and comprehensible to you, anything goes.

Find yourself a comfortable position. Before you start writing, bring your awareness to your body, and notice any bodily sensations that are arising. Be aware of where your body is in contact with the floor or the chair. Now, bring your awareness to the natural flow of your breath. The trick with this meditation is to not to try too hard. It works best to divide your attention, focusing on the chosen focus (but not too intensely!) and keeping a background awareness of your body and breath as you write. When your mind wanders off, practice compassion, let go of self-criticism, and gently return your attention to the chosen focus. Notice and return.

Set your timer for 10 to 20 minutes … and … start writing. Keep your pen in contact with the paper and keep writing until your timer goes.

Write down whatever comes into your head. Your aim is to capture the stream of thoughts and feelings as they flow through your mind. Let go of your inner editor! Later, after the meditation has finished, you can read the writing and salvage those bits that are worth keeping, your gold, and discard the dross. However, for now just keep that pen moving and keep getting those thoughts down on paper. If your mind wanders too far off from your chosen focus, notice that and gently bring it back to the topic in hand.

As in the previous meditation, be aware of the physical act of writing and how it feels to be someone sitting here writing. Relax any parts of your body that do not need to be engaged with the act of writing. If you find that you are tensing up, slow your writing down, consciously relax, and reconnect with the flow of your breath. At the same time, keep writing! A relaxed attitude will help you access your subconscious mind, and it is here that we uncover our gold.

However, it's no problem if you find it impossible to relax—just keep on writing anyway. Part of your meditation can be to write and at the same time maintain a gentle awareness of how it feels to be tense, noticing sensations as they arise in your body. If you can't let it go, then just let it be.

Once your timer goes, put your pen down. Notice how your body feels, how you are feeling in yourself, and the natural flow of your breath. Be aware of where your body is in contact with the floor or your chair. And when you are ready, carry on with your day.

If you wish to, you can read the writing through immediately after the meditation. You might want to underline any sentences that strike you as interesting and worth pursuing. Or you might prefer to read the writing through later and sift through it to see if you can uncover any hidden gems.

Protecting Your Privacy

A young friend confided in me that because she lives in shared accommodation, she doesn't feel secure to put her thoughts down on paper in case one of her flatmates might read what she's written. Instead, she prefers to write digitally and keep her writing in a file with a secure password. It is understandable to feel concerned about privacy. You'll feel more liberated to express your true thoughts and feelings if you are certain that you've established a safe, private place to keep them.

When we practice writing meditation, we are writing for ourselves. Writing meditation is not about being nice; it is about being authentic. We give ourselves space to explore through our writing whatever crazy ideas our minds come up with, as some of these bizarre ideas can turn out to be pure genius. This can feel dangerous if you are uncertain whether you can protect your privacy. In order to feel safe to open your heart onto paper, you will need to consider how you are going to protect your writing from unwelcome attention. I am certain that as a creative person, you'll find ways to put boundaries up to protect your writing, until you are ready to share it with others.

This morning, in preparation for writing this chapter, I did a period of writing meditation. I wrote twelve pages, and afterward I tore up and composted eleven of those pages. I only felt the need to save one of the pages, as it contained lots of useful ideas for this chapter. All the pages were of value, as they helped me clear my head of all the detritus that gets in the way of clear writing. However, I am not precious about my writing meditation writing. I am genuinely more interested in the process than I am in the outcome, so I don't mind letting go of most of the writing. I find that following a period of meditative writing, when I sit at the computer to write, my writing is fresher, flows more easily, and is more inspired.

However, it can be interesting to keep a copy of your writing, especially when you are first starting out. It's informative every so often to look back over what you've written, noticing what's changed and how you have grown and developed. For privacy you could keep your writing under lock and key or store it digitally as my friend does. Sometimes if some of the writing I've done during writing meditation really shines, then I scan a copy of it and store it in a computer file. I write on lose file paper rather than in a notebook, so it makes it easy to tear a page out to scan or to compost. The other advantage of storing it in this way is that it can be easily found without searching through mountains of notebooks.

How to Use the Chakra Meditation Questions

Each of the chakra chapters concludes with a set of meditation questions related to the chakra's themes. Working with these questions will help you explore the theme, gain insights relevant to your own life, and bring about transformation and healing.

The meditation questions are simple to use and can easily be fitted into your day. They are a way of accessing your own inner life coach and help you gain access to the wisdom of your subconscious. They build your confidence in your ability to create positive change in your life.

To give you an idea of how to use the meditation questions, let's have a look at one. For example, in the root chakra chapter, we are developing the theme of building a stable base to support our creativity. One of the meditation questions in this chapter is "Which activities do I find grounding and help create stability in my life?" You could work with this question in the following ways:

- In the evening at bedtime pose the question, and then overnight let your subconscious mind get to work on coming up with some answers to it.
- Pose the question while out walking or during a walking meditation. Gently turn the question over in your mind; you don't need to chase the answers.

- Use the question as your focus during a sitting meditation. If your mind wanders off, gently bring it back to the question and your mind's response to it.
- Use the question as your focus for a writing meditation. Set your timer for 5 to 20 minutes and just write down whatever comes into your head in response to the question. No need to worry about spelling, grammar, handwriting, and so on. Just keep the pen on the paper and keep writing.
- Pose the question at the beginning or end of your yoga session during a period of relaxation. Or repeat it silently while you are holding a yoga pose and relaxing into it.

Whichever way you choose to use the meditation questions, be prepared for chakra rainbow magic to illuminate your life!

Also, remember to check out the chakra-inspired writing suggestions in each of the chakra chapters.

Writing to Heal Trauma

Journaling, or expressive writing, can be especially therapeutic for those with a history of trauma. Research has shown that writing can help with processing traumatic events and can "reduce the severe symptoms that can accompany trauma," eventually helping the sufferer rediscover the positive aspects of life again, writes research scientist Courtney Ackerman in an online article. "Writing works to enhance our mental health through guiding us towards confronting previously inhibited emotions (reducing the stress from inhibition), helping us process difficult events and compose a coherent narrative about our experiences, and possibly even through repeated exposure to the negative emotions associated with traumatic memories."[20]

My own personal experience of recovering from trauma has taught me that when traumatic experiences are repressed, they block the free flow of energy and sap our creativity. Conversely, my own journey has shown me that it is possible to use a creative approach to map out a path of recovery that will ultimately lead you to a sense of wholeness and healing again.

As I mentioned at the start of this chapter, in 2020 both my parents died within a few weeks of each other. I experienced a tsunami of grief, and as a survivor of childhood abuse, my grieving process was complicated and messy. At times I felt overwhelmed,

---

20. Ackerman, "83 Benefits of Journaling for Depression, Anxiety, and Stress."

and in normal times I would have sought professional help from a trained counsellor. However, these were not normal times. It was a pandemic, and here in the UK we had just gone into the first of several lockdowns. Due to the pandemic, face-to-face counselling was not available, and I did not want to have online or telephone counseling because what I had to discuss was so sensitive. At the time I had a strong sense that if I was going to be able to move forward with my life, now was the right time to deal with the waves of troubling feelings that were arising, and so I decided to devise my own program for processing and healing the trauma.

I am sharing my story of how I dealt with the trauma here, because I think it might be helpful for those of you in similar situations. However, if you are recovering from trauma, I recommend that it might be safer and less overwhelming for you to initially seek professional help to assist you on your healing journey, rather than trying to tackle it alone with self-help methods.

The two books that helped me most and acted as my support during this period were *Your Turn for Care: Surviving the Aging and Death of the Adults Who Harmed You* by Laura S. Brown, PhD, and *Overcoming Childhood Trauma: A Self-Help Guide Using Cognitive Behavioural Techniques* by Helen Kennerley. In many ways lockdown was the perfect time to do this sort of self-directed therapy work, as I was not teaching, so I was free to devote two weeks to the healing process of recovering from trauma. Over those two weeks I systematically worked my way through the CBT exercises in *Overcoming Childhood Trauma*. The CBT exercises involved systematically revisiting, and picturing in minute details, the traumatic events of my childhood.

I supplemented the CBT exercises with walking meditation, writing meditation, and the Working with Difficult Feelings mindfulness meditation, which augmented and multiplied the benefits of the CBT therapy and helped me recover more speedily from the effects of reliving the trauma. The methods I used are listed below:

> *Yoga:* I found physical yoga practice was an excellent way to release the memory of the trauma, which had been stored for years in my muscles as tension. While I was doing the two weeks of self-directed CBT therapy, which involved reliving in my mind the trauma I endured as a child, I found I experienced a lot of unpleasant physical tension, including tension headaches. Yoga practice was a wonderful antidote to this tension and allowed me to let go of and release both the difficult emotions and the physical residual tension.

Walking Meditation: Like many people who have been abused during childhood, I tend to disassociate when I remember what happened to me. The CBT therapy I used involved a technique of remembering the traumatic experiences in as much sensory detail as possible. The reasoning behind this is that repeated exposure to the feelings brought up by thinking about the event reduces the intensity of their impact. I found the best way to relive traumatic events from my childhood and avoid zoning out was to remember and picture the events while doing a walking meditation, and in this way I was grounding myself as I walked and remembered.

Writing Meditation: I mostly used the Writing Meditation with Focus (see page 44) to process the therapy I was doing. I would usually precede the writing meditation with a walking meditation as described earlier. Yesterday, in preparation for writing this section of the book, I reread the writing I did last year during that period of self-directed trauma therapy. Reading back reminded me of all the useful lessons that I had learned from doing the writing and therapy. It also reminded me of the coping skills that I had discovered through the process of doing the therapy, which will continue to be useful to me as I continue my recovery. Writing is such a powerful activity to do for someone who has suffered abuse, because while the abuse was done to you and you had no control over it, writing, on the other hand, empowers you to create your own narrative and enables you to exit a negative downward spiral and emerge renewed and with hope.

The Surrounding a Difficulty with Love Meditation: I used this mindfulness meditation anytime I got overwhelmed by difficult feelings. It's a very simple meditation in which you bring to mind something that is troubling you, notice how it manifests in your body as tightness or tension, and surround the corresponding area with love. I used an audio version of this meditation.[21] I think when you are meditating upon difficult feelings, it is good to be talked through the meditation, as then you get a sense of being supported.

---

21. Lizabeth Roemer and Susan M. Orsillo, "Inviting a Difficulty in and Working It Through the Body," Mindful Way Through Anxiety, 2014, https://mindfulwaythroughanxiety.com/exercises/.

Mindfulness of Body and Breath: I find this popular mindfulness meditation is excellent to bring you firmly back into your body after working with traumatic issues. I use an audio version, read by Mark Williams, and his reassuring voice always makes me feel comforted, safe, and looked after.[22]

The Four-Minute Check-In Meditation: This is my version of the popular mindfulness meditation, the Three-Minute Breathing Space.[23] It's good to practice it regularly, as then the skills are in place when you need to use them for emergency emotional first aid. It is simple, short, and hugely effective. In step 1 of the meditation, you tune in to your thoughts, feelings, and bodily sensations; in step 2 you center yourself; and then in step 3 you widen your awareness out again. It's a perfect way to ground and align yourself when you have been thrown off course by events.

Working with the Chakras: My experience has taught me that an awareness of the chakras is very helpful when recovering from trauma, especially working with the first four chakras, as they help you build strong foundations, find support, establish boundaries, build healthy relationships, reconnect with what gives you pleasure, connect with your loving heart, and open up to the possibility of forgiveness.

I am sharing the story of my recovery from trauma with you because I think it is a strong testimony to the healing power of yoga, walking meditation, writing meditation, and mindfulness. If your trauma has healed to the point that you feel safe and able to work without a therapist, then you might wish to explore the methods suggested here and use your powers of creativity to devise your own self-help program. However, please do treat yourself with kindness and compassion, acknowledging if you are not yet ready to face this healing journey alone.

Although the healing process I went through last year was painful, I did not at any point feel that I was in too deep or overwhelmed, mainly because I have many years of yoga practice behind me, and I am practiced at using mindfulness meditation to work with difficult emotions. Also, in the past, I have had counseling about my childhood, so

---

22. Mark Williams and Danny Penman, "Mindfulness Meditation of Body and Breath," Mindfulness: Finding Peace in a Frantic World, 2022, http://franticworld.com/free-meditations-from-mindfulness/.

23. Mark Williams and Danny Penman, "Three-Minute Breathing Space," Mindfulness: Finding Peace in a Frantic World, 2022, http://franticworld.com/free-meditations-from-mindfulness/.

I had already processed some of the past events in a supportive environment. I am also super lucky to have an exceptionally loving and supportive husband who knows about and understands what I went through in my childhood. Your situation might be quite different, so please do not feel that you must go it alone.

My two weeks of self-directed trauma recovery therapy were intense. At the time, my husband was off work and at home due to the pandemic. I half jokingly warned him that if he came across me walking and weeping, not to worry and that I was okay! And it was true: although I cried a lot during that time, they were healing tears, and I always felt able to cope. It was hard at times remembering painful events, but I always knew that my practice was there for me. The years of yoga, walking meditation, writing meditation, and mindfulness stood me in good stead and were there for me when I really needed them. And hugs from my lovely husband, Simon, as well of course!

On the night I finished doing my CBT therapy, I dreamed that I returned to the street where I had lived as a child. In front of my childhood home was a skip filled with rubbish (which on awaking I interpreted as being all the difficult feelings I was processing and letting go of). Then, in the dream, I noticed a gap between two of the houses that had not been there before, revealing a beautiful piece of land where flowers grew and an orchard was in blossom. In the dream I turned to my husband and said, "Well, there's a plot that's ripe for building on." The dream seemed to answer a question that I had been asking myself, which was "Can I create anything beautiful out of this?" The dream seemed to confirm that yes, it would be possible to derive sweetness from all these bitter ingredients. It revealed to me that despite the traumatic nature of my childhood, underneath all the pain and hurt, there remains intact a wholeness and a wild beauty that I can build upon.

A Word to Would-Be Writers

Whatever creative discipline you are working in, the writing meditation techniques described in this chapter will help you to access your inner wisdom, shift creative blocks, and generate ideas. However, I often get mail from readers of my books who feel they have a book in them and want to know how to go about getting published, so this section is for them.

The ideas we explored earlier in this chapter form an enjoyable and effective way of establishing a routine of writing. Using the writing meditation methods, you'll never be short of ideas. However, if you want to get published, then you will need to hone your writing skills so that you can produce something that is readable and that people want to read.

I'd been working for a few years on my first book, *Yoga Through the Year*, when it struck me that I didn't know how to write! Yes, I could string words together on paper and I had no shortage of ideas, but in order to convey my ideas more effectively, I needed to learn writing skills and master my craft. It was a humbling moment, and it did slow me down considerably as I set myself the task of completing a course on writing with the University of East Anglia. This paid off, as subsequently I started getting articles published in yoga magazines, and it eventually led to my first book, *Yoga Through the Year*, being accepted for publication!

It's fine to be experimental in your writing, but you'll be a better communicator if you've taken the time to learn your craft. Of course, this applies to all the creative disciplines. For example, take the artist Picasso. His work is pure iconoclastic genius, but it only works because he knew the rules of drawing and painting and so he could confidently break them.

Learning your craft doesn't need to be arduous. If you love writing, painting, baking, or sculpting, learning the skills of your craft can be a joy. The thing I love about both yoga and writing is that there's always more to learn. It gives me such pleasure when I come across a new way of combining yoga poses into a novel, delicious, flowing sequence. Likewise, to write well you have to be a good reader, and reading innovative, surprising new writing will inspire you to reach higher with your own work.

Like a garden, writing practice is never finished. There is always more to learn, but it's a wonderful journey, and along the way you'll learn so much and meet some wonderful people. For ideas on creative writing courses and books, check out the resources section at the end of this book.

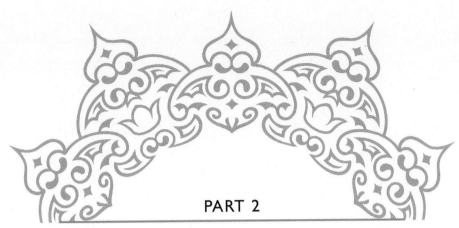

PART 2

The Chakras for Creativity

CHAPTER 5

Root Chakra
(Muladhara)

Build Strong Foundations for Your Creativity

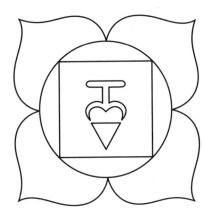

Root Chakra Symbol

This blood-red chakra provides a solid foundation for your creativity. When you work with this chakra, you learn to take care of your basic survival needs, leaving you free to build up your creativity from a secure and solid base. With the earth supporting you, you can put down roots and your creativity can grow and be sustained. This is the place where your creativity finds a home.

The Root Chakra at a Glance

Sanskrit Name: *Muladhara* (root or support)

Physical Location: The base of the spine, the pelvic floor, the legs, and the feet

Element: Earth

Color: Red

Yantra: Square

Seed Mantra: Lam (pronounced *lum*)

Affirmations: *The earth supports me. The earth nourishes me.*

Main Creative Concerns: Developing a stable base to create from and attending to the practical details, which enable us to lead a creative, fulfilled life.

Balanced: Basic human needs are met, creating a sense of emotional and physical stability. Feels connected to and supported by others. Grounded. Comfortable in one's own skin. At home in the world.

Excessive: Over concern with the material side of life, to the detriment of more spiritual concerns. Fixated on security. Inability to take risks or to tolerate the chaos of the creative process.

Deficient: Neglects basic needs and is rootless. Chaotic lifestyle. Ungrounded, emotionally and physically unstable. Airy-fairy, impractical, lives in head, dis-association, out of body sensations.

Life Issues: Ensuring basic human needs for food, shelter, and protection are met. Sexuality. Finding your tribe. Resolving family issues. Feeling comfortable in your own skin and assured of your place in the world.

Healing Practices: Nest building, gardening, cooking, DIY, household management (paying bills on time, keeping your house in order), healing family rifts, forgiveness, healing childhood traumas, making a family tree, finding out about your ancestors, connecting with like minds, finding your tribe, being in nature, pets, self-care, reflexology, yoga, dancing, walking, cycling, environmental activism, making things with your hands, creative activities.

Creating Order out of Chaos

Your creative practice needs strong roots if it is to grow and flourish. In this chapter we will be considering what we need to do to establish firm foundations for our creativity. Human beings have a basic need to be creative and express themselves, and even in incredibly challenging situations the beauty of the human spirit will oftentimes find a way to rise above difficulties and create something of beauty. However, generally we are more likely to be able to get involved with creative activities if our basic human needs for shelter, food, warmth, and human connection are met.

Creativity is a subversive activity; it is going against the norm, as society favors more functional, practical activities. When you first start living more creatively, you might come up against both internal and external resistance to doing so. You might ask yourself why you are writing, sewing, painting, or doing any other creative pursuit when there are so many more practical jobs that need attending to. To be a woman and an artist is even more an act of subversion, as women have to overcome their conditioning that dictates that they should put taking care of everyone's practical needs before their own need for fulfillment.

For our creativity to flourish, there is a balance to be struck between attending to everyday needs and rising above the quotidian to express ourselves through whatever artistic medium we have chosen. Creativity enables us to create order from chaos, although sometimes, to pursue our creative pursuits, we must turn a blind eye to the chaos around us. Even though the house is dusty, the dishes need doing, and there is a mountain of laundry to fold, we still choose to spend time writing, painting, sculpting, or knitting.

To be creative it is essential to be able to tolerate a certain amount of chaos. Most creative projects begin with a chaotic phase, and it is out of this chaos that the creative process creates meaning and beauty. To be able to give the creative process the time and care it deserves, for a while you might have to turn a blind eye to disorder in order to see a project through to completion. However, if you neglect the everyday chores for too long, they might well end up disrupting your creative process and making it impossible for you to function.

I find one way around this conundrum is to use my best energy for writing, so I mostly do that in the morning. Later in the day I'll use my second-best energy for catching up with the practical tasks that when done make life run more smoothly.

However, everyday chores can also be a friend to creativity. I usually intersperse periods of writing with mindfully doing everyday tasks about the house. This benefits me because it means I have periods of activity, which prevents my job from being too sedentary, and it gets my blood flowing, which benefits my brain and thought process. If I am stuck, blocked, or confused about which way to go with an idea, I find doing some washing up, making the bed, or vacuuming will unblock me, and often an idea or the perfect solution just pops into my head as if by magic. The rhythmic nature of a mundane task is soothing and allows ideas to flow.

The root chakra is very much about keeping our house in order. This might also include attending to the practical details that will enable you to fulfill your creative dreams and potential, such as finding a space to work; carving out chunks of time; finding childcare if you have kids; keeping yourself fit, healthy, and well nourished; and having a tribe of people around you who understand and support your creative vision.

What Is Your Creation Story?

The root chakra is the doorway to the ancestors, and we heal this chakra when we connect with those who came before us. It is also important to look at and understand what your place was in your family of origin. Did you have a happy childhood? Were you wanted and loved? What is your creation story and how does it affect your ability to live creatively now?

I know from personal experience that the root chakra offers us a wonderful opportunity to heal trauma and frees us to creatively move forward with our life. As someone who suffered trauma and abuse in my childhood, for a large part of my life I have been someone without a story, or at least I had a story, but not one I felt able tell. When you are unable to tell your story, it's hard for people to understand where you're coming from. For example, my passion/obsession for empowering and protecting women from abuse makes more sense when you consider my father's coercive control over my mother. Likewise, I think it was hard for people to understand my past struggles with anxiety and just how much yoga had helped me find a more peaceful way of being. However, now that I am free to tell my story, I have made a conscious choice to only tell part of it, to protect both my own and other family members' privacy. Working with the chakras teaches us to protect our own and others' boundaries.

I made a conscious decision in my thirties not to cut off any members of my family of origin, even though contact with them was often intensely painful. I was influenced in this decision by Harriet Lerner's book, *The Dance of Anger*, in which she suggested that by cutting family members off you create a very intense relationship with them, whereas by maintaining some form of contact, even if it's minimal, you reduce the intensity of the relationship.[24] I have found that you can learn so much from all members of your family, whether you get on with them or not, if you are open to hearing their story. Even though you don't choose your family, if you take the time to hear the story that your blood relatives have to tell, you will learn so much about yourself and where you came from. And this is the healing work we have to do when we work with the root chakra.

I'd strongly recommend talking to older family members, as you can learn so much about your family's history in this way. Also, sometimes we uncover a mantle of suffering that has been handed down across the generations and is playing out in current family relations. The Buddhist monk Thich Nhat Hanh has created some beautiful meditations in which you send love, healing, and forgiveness to your parents, your ancestors, and of course yourself.[25]

However, if having contact with your family puts you in emotional or physical danger, there are lots of alternative ways that you can work with the root chakra to bring about transformation and healing. Any form of counseling in which you share and resolve past issues and hurts is healing for this chakra, and conversely, any work you do on the root chakra will support the therapeutic counseling process. Finding support is also a way of working on this chakra, so do reach out to others for help.

If, like me, you had instability in your early years, then you will find that it pays dividends to regularly return to working on the root chakra. Many creative people have had troubled childhoods, and although I would not wish an unhappy childhood on anyone, I can confirm that there are a multitude of healing practices that help us to find wholeness again. And we can retrieve our story and create something of beauty out of it.

Yoga Inspired by the Root Chakra

To create, we must first picture what we wish to create; this involves a lot of abstract thinking, which can leave us feeling stuck in our head and ungrounded. Working on a creative project can become all-consuming, and even when you're not working on the project you find yourself still thinking about it. This might just be a sign that you're fully engaged with the work, which is fine. However, when engagement with your work tips into obsession, you can end up feeling distracted and ungrounded, living in your head, and find yourself problem-solving in the early hours of the morning when you'd rather be asleep. And then

---

24. Harriet Lerner, *The Dance of Anger: A Woman's Guide to Changing the Patterns of Intimate Relationships* (London: HarperCollins UK, 2004), 196.

25. Nhat Hanh, Thich, *Reconciliation: Healing the Inner Child* (Berkeley, CA: Parallax Press, 2010), 65–70.

those around you suffer because you are not fully present when you're with them. Working with the root chakra, *muladhara,* is the perfect antidote to this spaciness and will bring you back into your body again and bring you back down to earth with a soft landing!

Once you are back in your body, your creations are more likely to become embodied, rather than being just great ideas stuck in your head. Also, when you are grounded—that is, you are connected to and supported by the earth beneath you—then you are more likely to feel physically, mentally, and emotionally stable, which is a much better place to create from.

The root chakra is associated with the lower parts of the body, the pelvic floor, the legs, and the feet, so when we are designing a root chakra–inspired yoga practice, we focus on this area. One way to ground yourself is to simply bring your attention to these parts of the body. If you are sitting, become aware of where your body is in contact with the floor, your chair, or your support. If you are standing, then become aware of where your feet are in contact with and supported by the earth beneath you.

Great poses for grounding are Mountain Pose (*Tadasana*), all versions of Warrior Pose (*Virabhadrasana*), Tree Pose (*Vrksasana*), and most of yoga's standing poses. You could also work with yoga sequences (*vinyasas*) such as Salute to the Moon (*Chandra Namaskar*), Salute to the Sun (*Surya Namaskar*), or Bow to the Earth (*Bhumi Pranam*).

When working with this chakra, you could also include elements such as flower imagery, the color red, the seed mantra *Lam*, and the earth element.

Root Chakra Yoga Practice

The Root Chakra Yoga Practice is grounding, gently energizing, calming, nurturing, and induces a sense of peacefulness. It will help you to develop your creative focus and help you to feel supported in your creative endeavors.

The affirmations we use in the practice are *The earth supports me* and *The earth nourishes me.* They can be coordinated with the breath:

Inhale: The earth supports me.

Exhale: The earth nourishes me.

Allow 20 to 30 minutes.

At the end of these instructions, you'll find an illustrated aide-mémoire for the whole practice.

1. Root Chakra Awareness Exercise, lying on back, with knees bent and feet on floor

Close your eyes. Notice where your body is touching the floor or your support. Feel yourself relaxing into the support of the earth beneath you. Now bring your awareness to the area between the base of the spine and the pubic bone. Notice how with each inhalation and exhalation there is a corresponding movement in this area.

Now, silently repeat the root chakra affirmation, coordinating it with the breath. Inhale and affirm, *The earth supports me.* Exhale and affirm, *The earth nourishes me.*

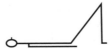

Relaxation Pose, lying on back, with knees bent and feet on floor

2. Leg Stretch Sequence

Bring both knees onto your chest. Inhale and straighten your legs vertically, heels toward the ceiling, and take your arms out to the side just below shoulder height, palms facing up. Exhale and bring your knees back to your chest and hands back to your knees. Next time around, inhale, straighten your legs vertically, and take your arms over your head and onto the floor behind you. On each inhale affirm, *The earth supports me.* And on each exhale affirm, *The earth nourishes me.* Repeat the sequence 6 times, alternating arm movements.

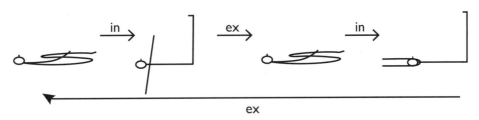

Leg Stretch Sequence

3. Cat Pose (*Marjaryasana*) into Child's Pose (*Balasana*)

Come onto all fours. Exhaling, round the back into Cat Pose (*Marjaryasana*) and lower the bottom to the heels and the head to the floor into Child's Pose (*Balasana*). Inhaling, come back up to all fours. Repeat 6 times. On each exhale, silently repeat the mantra *Lam* (pronounced *lum*).

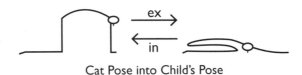

Cat Pose into Child's Pose

4. Mountain Pose (*Tadasana*)

Stand tall, with feet parallel and about hip width apart. Be aware of the contact between your feet and the earth beneath you. Imagine a string attached to the crown of your head, gently pulling you skyward; simultaneously, let your tailbone drop and feel your heels rooting down into the earth. On each inhale affirm, *The earth supports me*. And on each exhale affirm, *The earth nourishes me*.

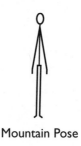

Mountain Pose

5. Bend and straighten warm-up, with mantra *Lam*

Take the legs 2 to 3 feet apart and turn the toes slightly out. Take the arms out to the sides at shoulder height, palms facing downward. On your next exhale, bend the knees and lower the arms, chanting aloud the mantra *Lam*. Inhale, returning to the starting position. Repeat 8 times.

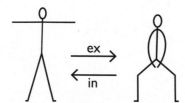

Bend and straighten warm-up

6. Tree Pose (*Vrksasana*)

Stand tall, feet hip width apart, hands in Prayer Position (*Namaste*). Imagine that like a tree, you have roots going from the soles of your feet way down into the earth. Then bring the sole of your right foot to rest on your inner left thigh, rotating your right knee out to the side. Either keep your hands at the heart or take your arms above the head, hands in Prayer Position. Fix your gaze on a point that is not moving. Stay for a few breaths. Repeat on the other side.

For balance problems, instead of bringing the foot onto the thigh, just rest the sole of the foot on the opposite inside ankle or be near a wall for support.

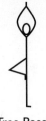

Tree Pose

7. Albatross Sequence 1

Stand tall, with feet hip width apart. Inhaling, raise the arms above the head. Exhaling, bend forward about 45 degrees with your back slightly arched and arms spread out to the sides like a bird's wings (this is Albatross Pose). Stay for one breath in the pose. Inhaling, come back up to standing, sweeping the arms above the head. Exhaling, lower the arms back to the sides. Repeat the sequence 4 to 6 times.

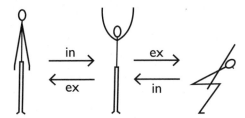

Albatross Sequence 1

8. Standing *Lam* Sequence

Stand in Mountain Pose (*Tadasana*) with hands in Prayer Position (*Namaste*). Inhale, raising the arms. Exhale, chanting aloud the mantra *Lam* and coming into a Standing Forward Bend (*Uttanasana*). Inhale, taking the arms up above the head as you come back up to standing. Exhale, silently chanting the mantra *Lam*, coming into a Half-Squat (*Utkatasana* variation), thighs parallel to the floor and hands touching the floor (if possible). Inhale, coming back up to standing and taking the arms above the head. Exhale, lowering the arms, coming back into Mountain Pose, hands together in prayer.

Repeat the sequence 4 to 6 times.

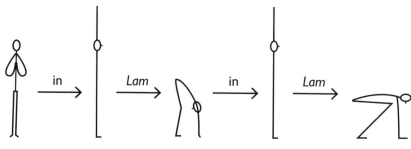

Standing *Lam* Sequence

9. Floor Salute to the Sun (*Surya Namaskar* variation)

Come to tall kneeling, hands in Prayer Position (*Namaste*). Inhale, raising both arms above your head. Exhale, folding forward into Child's Pose (*Balasana*). Inhale, coming onto all fours, and turning the toes under; exhaling, push into Downward-Facing Dog Pose (*Adho Mukha Svanasana*).

Then go back through the sequence in reverse order. Inhale, back onto all fours. Exhale into Child's Pose. Inhale, coming back up to tall kneeling and arms above the head; exhale, lower the arms, hands into Prayer Position.

Repeat the sequence 4 to 6 times. (If you prefer, it's fine to ignore the breathing guidance that's given for this sequence. Take extra breaths if you need to. Never strain with the breathing.)

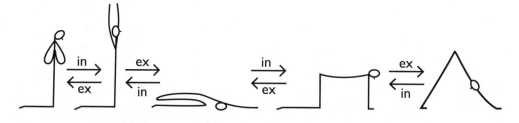

Floor Salute to the Sun

10. Supine Twist (*Jathara Parivrtti*)

Lie on your back, knees bent, feet together, arms out to the sides at shoulder height, and palms facing down. Bring both knees onto your chest (for an easier pose keep both feet on the floor). Exhaling, lower both knees down toward the floor on the left and turn the head gently to the right. Inhale and return to center. Allow your movements to be flowing and watery. Repeat 6 times on each side, alternating sides.

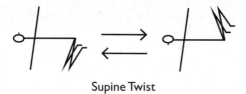

Supine Twist

11. Leg Stretch Sequence

We end the practice with the same sequence we began with, which gives a pleasing circular feel to the practice.

Bring both knees onto your chest. Inhale and straighten your legs vertically, heels toward the ceiling, and take your arms out to the side just below shoulder height, palms facing up. Exhale and bring your knees back to your chest and hands back to your knees. Next time around, inhale, straighten your legs vertically, and take your arms over your head and onto the floor behind you. On each inhale affirm, *The earth supports me.* And on each exhale affirm, *The earth nourishes me.* Repeat the sequence 6 times, alternating arm movements.

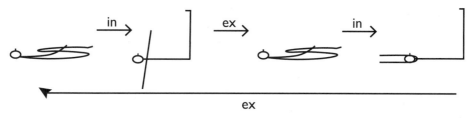

Leg Stretch Sequence

12. Short relaxation or Root Chakra Meditation

You can either finish your practice with a few minutes lying down in the Relaxation Pose (*Savasana*) or, if you have time, find a comfortable seated position and do the Root Chakra Meditation that follows this practice.

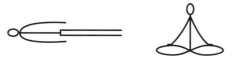

Short relaxation or Root Chakra Meditation

Root Chakra Yoga Practice Overview

1. Root Chakra Awareness Exercise

2. Leg Stretch Sequence × 6. Inhale: *The earth supports me.* Exhale: *The earth nourishes me.*

3. Cat Pose into Child's Pose with silent mantra *Lam* × 6

4. Mountain Pose. Inhale: *The earth supports me.* Exhale: *The earth nourishes me.*

5. Bend and straighten warm-up with mantra *Lam* × 8

6. Tree Pose

7. Albatross Sequence 1 × 4–6

8. Standing *Lam* Sequence × 4–6

9. Floor Salute to the Sun × 4–6

10. Supine Twist × 6 each side

11. Leg Stretch Sequence × 6

12. Short relaxation or Root Chakra Meditation

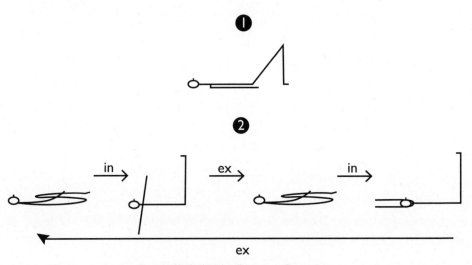

Root Chakra Yoga Practice Overview

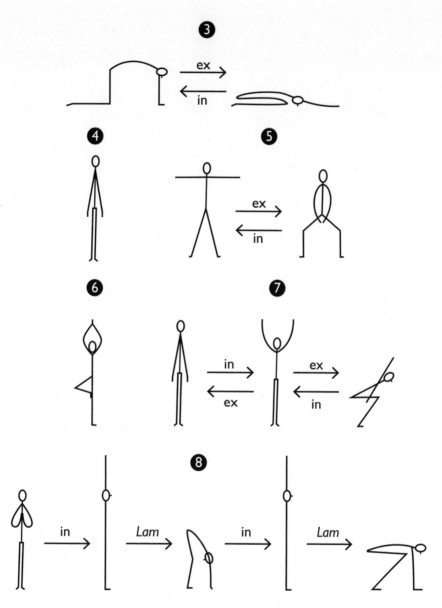

Root Chakra Yoga Practice Overview (continued)

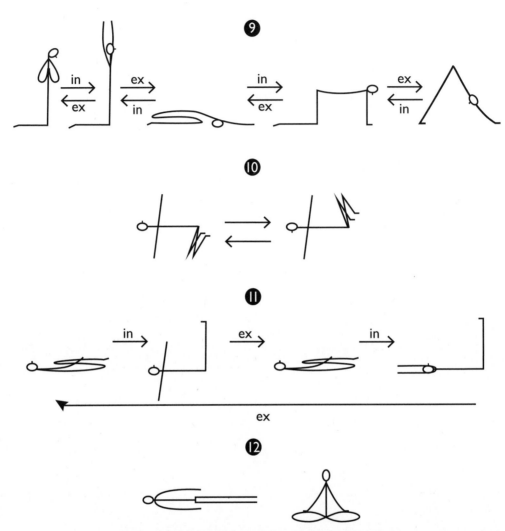

Root Chakra Yoga Practice Overview (continued)

MEDITATION
Root Chakra Meditation

You can use the Root Chakra Meditation to begin or end a yoga practice, or it can be used on its own as a standalone practice.

This meditation creates a sense of stability; quietens a fearful, anxious mind; and is calming. If you are feeling lonely or unsupported, it will help you feel nurtured and nourished. If you are feeling disassociated or ungrounded, it will help you to feel grounded and centered.

Find yourself a comfortable seated position. Bring your awareness to the pelvic floor, the area between the base of the spine and the pubic bone. Throughout the meditation, keep bringing your awareness back into this part of your body. Keep your awareness here and silently repeat the affirmation for the practice several times, coordinating it with the breath:

Inhale: The earth supports me.

Exhale: The earth nourishes me.

Then, let go of the affirmation, and keeping your awareness at the pelvic floor, visualize a red flower. Picture the color and shape of the flower. Notice whether it is open or in bud.

Now let go of the image of the flower and bring your awareness to the natural flow of your breath. As you breathe, rest your awareness at the pelvic floor, and notice how there is a gentle movement here that corresponds with the rhythm of the breath. With each inhale there is a slight downward pressure on the pelvic floor, and with each exhale there is a slight contraction. With each exhalation gently pull the pelvic floor muscles in and up, and with each inhalation relax these muscles. Then, once you have established this rhythm, begin on each exhale to silently repeat the mantra *Lam* (pronounced *lum*). Repeat the mantra several times.

After several silent repetitions, begin to chant the mantra *Lam* aloud several times. As you chant keep your awareness at the pelvic floor and the lower part of the body.

When you feel ready, let go of chanting. Enjoy the silence for a few breaths. Notice how you feel now at the end of your Root Chakra Meditation. Once again become aware of where your body is in contact with the floor or support. Take this grounded, centered feeling into the next thing that you do today.

MEDITATION
Root Chakra Walking Meditation

Walking of any sort is beneficial to the root chakra. It is grounding and strengthens your connection with your surroundings and with the earth. It calms and clears the mind, helping relieve and release stress, gently boosting the circulation and putting a smile back on your face!

You can practice this simple root chakra walking meditation anytime you have to walk anywhere, from the car to your house, up or down stairs, along a corridor at work, in the park, or in your garden. The beauty of it is that it can easily be fitted into even the busiest of days.

In this walking meditation you simply pay attention to how it feels to walk, noticing any sensations you experience in the feet as you walk. How does it feel as you lift your foot, and how does it feel as your foot makes contact with the earth again? Be aware of the contact that your feet are making with the earth beneath you and how the earth supports you.

When I am doing this root chakra walking meditation, I like to repeat the phrase "Kiss the earth with your feet." This is the instruction on walking meditation given by the Buddhist monk Thich Nhat Hanh in his poem *Walking Meditation*, and in the poem, he shows us how to walk in a way that generates the energy of peacefulness and happiness.[26]

MEDITATION
Root Chakra Writing Meditation

For full instructions on how to do a writing meditation, go to the Writing Meditation with Focus section (page 44). Set your timer for 10 to 20 minutes and write meditatively on one or more of the following subjects:

- Earth
- Red
- Home

---

26. Nguyen Ahn-Huong and Thich Nhat Hanh, *Walking Meditation* (Boulder, CO: Sounds True, 2006), 6–7.

- Family
- Finding my tribe

If writing isn't your thing, feel free to work with the above topics in other mediums. For example, paint a picture, make a collage, compose a song, or take some photos, working with the theme: earth, red, home, and so on.

Root Chakra Meditation Questions

For full instructions on how to use the meditation questions, see page 47.

- What practical steps do I need to take to create the time and space needed for my creative pursuits?
- What is my creative lineage and who from this lineage inspires my work?
- What are the creative heirlooms/talents that I have inherited from my ancestors?
- Which activities do I find grounding and help create stability in my life?
- Who supports my creativity and how can I show my gratitude to them?

CHAPTER 6

Sacral Chakra
(Svadhisthana)

Creativity That Flows from the Center

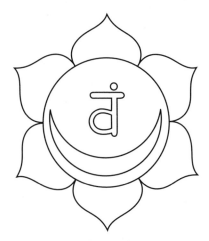

Sacral Chakra Symbol

Working with this watery chakra teaches you to ride the ebb and flow of your creativity. This juicy orange chakra picks you up and carries you on a wave of pleasure, and through your work, you get to share that pleasure with others. The sacral chakra links your creativity to the umbilical cord of life, you learn about the attraction of opposites, and your ideas are fertilized and grow.

The Sacral Chakra at a Glance

Sanskrit Name: Svadhisthana (one's own abode, sweetness)

Physical Location: The navel, the belly, lower abdomen, and areas of the body associated with sexual pleasure and procreation

Element: Water

Color: Orange

Yantra: Upward-pointing crescent moon

Seed Mantra: Vam (pronounced *vum*)

Affirmations: I trust myself. My inner wisdom guides me.

Main Creative Concerns: Riding the ebb and flow of creativity. Seeking and giving pleasure through your work.

Balanced: A good sense of self, healthy boundaries, fulfilling relationships, open to giving and receiving pleasure, at ease with sexuality, creative, emotionally intelligent, able to ride the ebb and flow of life.

Excessive: Poor boundaries, no sense of self, dependency, addictive tendencies, sexually reckless, manic, irrational, ruled by emotions, uncentered, and self-destructive.

Deficient: In a rut, feeling stuck, out of touch with emotions, hyper-rational, lack of intuition, living in one's head, self-contained, sexually repressed, a drudge, cut off from pleasures of life.

Life Issues: Relationships, establishing healthy boundaries, seeking pleasure, finding enjoyment in life, sexuality, procreation, biorhythms, creativity.

Healing Practices: Socializing, healthy sexual relationships; being nurtured and nurturing; rhythmic physical activities, such as flowing yoga sequences, walking, running, cycling, swimming, belly dancing, tai chi, being near water, touching and being touched, breath awareness, and all creative activities.

Connecting with Your Creative Source

In the last chapter we thought about how we go about establishing roots for our creativity. In this chapter we will consider how to get our creativity flowing. The sacral chakra is the door to intuition and the flow of creation. Within each of us there is immensely more creative potential than we actually use. Yoga enables us to dive deep within ourselves and uncover our full creative potential. We do this by centering ourselves and tapping into an unlimited flow of creative energy.

You began life in your mother's womb. Life flowed into you through the umbilical cord, which supplied you with all the nourishment that you needed to develop and grow. The space at the navel, where as a baby you were connected to the stream of life, is a sacred place and a source of spiritual power. However, for many of us this center gets blocked by shame about the belly. Women in particular are conditioned to keep their belly pulled in tightly like a corset, which inhibits the breathing and the flow of energy. Yoga teaches us to develop a strong but supple core, establishing a healthy breathing pattern and connecting us through our sacral chakra to the stream of life.

If we want our creativity to flourish, we must nurture it like a mother nourishing her baby in the womb. We connect it to the flow of life, which gives us an unlimited source of creative potential to draw from. By dropping your awareness down into your belly, which is also the location of the sacral chakra, you can connect to a powerhouse of stored energy. Your yoga practice teaches you how to prevent your vital energy (*prana*) from becoming depleted and keeps this energy flowing. Yoga breathing (*pranayama*) infuses you with the breath of life and teaches you to regulate your energy flow. Yoga relaxation enables your body and mind to rest, removing any blockages that impede the free flow of pranic energy.

When we are anxious or preoccupied, our energy tends to get stuck in our heads. At these times we feel cut off from the flow of life and our creative impulses are blocked. You can shift to a healthier flow of energy by dropping your awareness down from your head to your belly. This is what we call centering. When you are centered, you immediately feel calmer, more focused, and receptive to new ideas and solutions. By centering you come home to yourself, feel more self-assured, and are better able to generate ideas and take ownership of them. If you combine centering with grounding (as described in the previous chapter), you become a truly formidable creative powerhouse!

The process of centering, dropping our awareness down to our belly, also enables us to access a deep source of wisdom that resides in the belly. When we are centered, we are able to listen to and respond to our "gut feelings." Western science recognizes the possibility that our gut acts as a "second brain" that influences our physical and mental sense of well-being.[27] Intuition is an important part of the creative process: it helps us make leaps of faith with greater confidence, oftentimes with spectacular results.

---

27. Fernando Pagés Ruiz, "Forget Six-Pack Abs: What It Really Means to Have Strong Abs," Yoga Journal, August 28, 2007, https://www.yogajournal.com/teach/anatomy-yoga-practice/forget-six-pack-abs/.

Creativity Powered by Pleasure

Whereas the root chakra was concerned with the tribal energy of the group and meeting the basic needs of survival, the sacral chakra is concerned with the need to evolve beyond the group, developing a separate sense of self, forming relationships with others, and receiving and giving pleasure.

To form healthy relationships, we must be able to establish healthy boundaries. To form healthy boundaries in relationships, frequently ask yourself the following questions:

- What do I think?
- What do I feel?
- What do I want?
- What brings me pleasure?

These are also useful questions to ask at any stage in the creative process, as they will keep you on track and ensure that your creations reflect your authentic self. Seeking out pleasure is about saying *yes!* to life. To say yes to the flow of life and allow it to flow through us and our creations, we need to cultivate the self-awareness that enables us to know what we want to affirm in our lives.

Pleasure seeking is often considered a narcissistic activity; however, pleasure can also be a motivating force in regard to our creative output. If your work brings you joy, you will want to keep returning to it. If there is an element of bliss in your creative endeavors, then it will compensate for the inevitable hard work and drudgery that is required to see any project through to completion.

Sometimes attributed to Pablo Picasso, the saying "The meaning of life is to find your gift. The purpose of life is to give it away," reminds us that when we are creative, we become part of a virtuous circle in which we receive inspiration, and through our creations, we give back to the river of life. Our yoga practice teaches us about this circular flow of giving and receiving love. With each inhale we receive love, and we are literally inspired; with each exhale, we give back love to the world.

Yoga flows, empowers, unfolds, reveals. Creativity lifts you up and takes you out of your everyday, habitual, familiar life. Creativity is learning to trust life. Creativity is being authentic, expressing your truth, and following your vison. Yoga is letting go of what impedes you from being creative and living a creative life. Inhale to inspire, exhale to let go. Yoga connects you to your inner wisdom and a universal creative force or power.

To live a creative life is to live with passion. When we walk the path of creativity, we become passionate about forming relationship with our authentic self, our soul-self, the one who knows. When we have remembered who we are and what our purpose is in life, the seeds we plant will land on fertile soil. The song we sing will be one of beauty.

Yoga Inspired by the Sacral Chakra

The sacral chakra inspires us to cultivate a sweetness in our yoga practice, which coincides with the pleasure-seeking principle of this chakra. Of course, generally yoga requires us to apply ourselves and exercise a gentle discipline; however, if your yoga sessions are pleasurable and sweet, you will want to keep on coming back to your mat.

One sublime way of connecting with life's sweetness would be to try a chocolate meditation (I allow myself this meditation once a week—you *can* have too much of a good thing!). Visualizing the chakra's associated color orange adds a stimulating, joyful element to the practice.

Water is the element associated with the sacral chakra, and so we choose watery, fluid movements and flowing yoga sequences (*vinyasas*) such as Salute to the Moon (*Chandra Namaskar*) or Salute to the Sun (*Surya Namaskar*).

Riding the waves of the breath helps us connect with the ebb and flow of life, especially if we center our attention in the lower abdomen, which is the part of the body connected with this chakra. We can combine this breath awareness with using the chakra's seed mantra, *Vam* (pronounced *vum*), on the exhale or silently at the end of the exhale.

Another way to work with this chakra is through an intuitive yoga session. Step onto your yoga mat and let your intuition guide you through a session. Your intuition will be sharpened by spending some time at the start of the session grounding and centering yourself. Then throughout the session, keep dropping your awareness down into your belly, which is the home of the sacral chakra and your intuition. If you are a yoga teacher, you'll find that teaching in this intuitive way is amazingly powerful. During an intuitive session, continually tune in to your inner wisdom, as well as sensing the prevailing energy of the participants in the class. I find that I get really positive feedback from students after an intuitive yoga session, with students saying things like "How did you know? That was exactly what I needed!"

Another way of working with this chakra is to explore yoga's approach to sacred sexuality. At various times in our lives, we may or may not be in a sexual relationship; however, sensual enjoyment, or everyday ecstasy is always available to us, and we can always choose to mindfully use our five senses to appreciate the beauty of the world around us and so fall head over heels in love with life again.

Sacral Chakra Yoga Practice

This is the go-to practice if you feel blocked and want to get your creative juices flowing again. It shifts blocked energy and enables you to go with the ebb and flow of life. It is a centering practice that connects you to your inner wisdom.

The affirmations we use in the practice are *I trust myself* and *My inner wisdom guides me.* They can be coordinated with the breath:

Inhale: I trust myself.

Exhale: My inner wisdom guides me.

Allow 30 to 40 minutes.

At the end of these instructions, you'll find an illustrated aide-mémoire for the whole practice.

1. Sacral Chakra Awareness Exercise, lying on the back, with knees bent and feet on floor
Close your eyes and bring your awareness to the lower abdomen, the area between the top of the pubic bone and the navel, which is the part of the body associated with the sacral chakra. Keeping your awareness in the belly, visualize an orange flower. Picture the color and shape of the flower.

Now let go of picturing the flower and silently repeat the chakra's affirmation several times, coordinating it with the breath. Inhale and affirm, *I trust myself.* Exhale and affirm, *My inner wisdom guides me.*

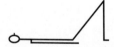

Relaxation Pose, lying on back, knees bent, feet on floor

2. Pelvic rocking
Lie on your back, both knees bent and both feet on the floor, about hip width apart. Notice the wavelike quality of the ebb and flow of your breath. Gently rock your pelvis back and forth. Exhale, tucking the tailbone under, as the back of the waist imprints into

the floor and the lower abs contract. Inhale, your tailbone rocking toward the floor, the back of the waist arching up away from the floor, and the tummy sticking out. Continue gently rocking between these two movements. Cultivate a wavelike quality to the movement and coordinate it with the breath.

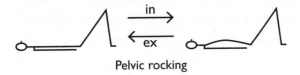

Pelvic rocking

3. Pelvic rocking and arm movements

Continue gently rocking your pelvis back and forth, and as you inhale, raise both arms above your head onto the floor behind you. As you exhale, lower the arms back to the sides. You can silently coordinate the breath and movement with the affirmation. Inhale and affirm, *I trust myself.* Exhale and affirm, *My inner wisdom guides me.* Repeat 6 times.

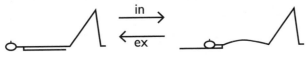

Pelvic rocking and arm movements

4. Supine Twist (*Jathara Parivrtti*)

Lie on your back, knees bent, feet together, arms out to the sides at shoulder height, and palms facing down. Bring both knees onto your chest (for an easier pose keep both feet on the floor). Exhaling, lower both knees down toward the floor on the left, and turn the head gently to the right. Inhale and return to center. With each exhale silently repeat the mantra *Vam* (pronounced *vum*). Allow your movements to be flowing and watery. Repeat 6 times on each side, alternating sides.

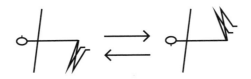

Supine Twist

5. Bridge Pose (*Setu Bandhasana*) into Knees-to-Chest Pose (*Apanasana*)

Lie on your back, knees bent, feet on the floor hip width apart, and arms by your sides. Inhaling, peel your back from the floor, taking your arms overhead onto the floor behind you, coming into Bridge Pose. Exhaling, lower the back, returning the arms back to the sides. Still exhaling (or take an extra breath), bring the knees to the chest and the hands to the knees, curling up into a ball, into Knees-to-Chest Pose. Inhale and come back to the starting position. Stay for one breath and then repeat the entire sequence. Aim to cultivate a wavelike quality to your movements, coordinating them with the breath. Repeat 4 to 6 times.

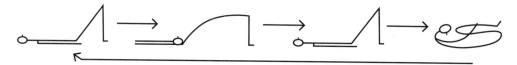

Bridge Pose into Knees-to-Chest Pose

6. Kneeling *Vam* Sequence

Come to tall kneeling, hands in the Prayer Position (*Namaste*). Inhale, raising both arms above your head. Exhale, chanting Vam (pronounced *vum*) aloud as you fold forward into Child's Pose (*Balasana*). From Child's Pose, inhale, coming into Upward-Facing Dog Pose (*Urdhva Mukha Svanasana*). Exhale back into Child's Pose. Inhale, coming back up to tall kneeling and moving arms above the head; exhale, lowering the arms, hands moving into Prayer Position.

Repeat the sequence 4 to 6 times. (If you prefer, it's fine to ignore the breathing guidance that's given for this sequence. Take extra breaths if you need to. Never strain with the breathing.)

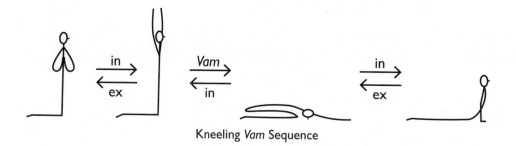

Kneeling *Vam* Sequence

7. Seated Twist variation (*Ardha Matsyendrasana*)

Come to a seated position, legs outstretched. Bend your right knee and place your right foot on the outside of your left knee. Sit up tall, wrap your left arm around your right knee, and hug the knee into your chest. Place your right hand, palm down, on the floor behind you. Inhale, lengthening up through your spine. Exhale and twist, looking over your right shoulder. Stay in the twist, dropping your awareness down to your belly. Each time you exhale, gently pull in your lower abs and silently repeat the mantra *Vam*. Stay for a few breaths and then repeat on the other side.

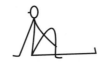

Seated Twist variation

8. Seated Forward Bend (*Paschimottanasana*)

Sit tall, with the legs outstretched (bend the knees to ease the pose). Inhale and raise your arms. Exhale and fold forward over the legs. Inhale and return to starting position. You can silently coordinate the breath and movement with the affirmation. Inhale and affirm, *I trust myself.* Exhale and affirm, *My inner wisdom guides me.* Repeat 6 times, and on the final time stay for a few breaths in the pose.

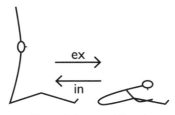

Seated Forward Bend

9. Supine Twist (*Jathara Parivrtti*)

Lie on your back, knees bent, feet together, arms out to the sides at shoulder height, and palms facing down. Bring both knees onto your chest. Exhale and lower both knees down toward the floor on the left. Stay here and place your left hand on your right thigh, gently persuading your legs down toward the floor. Turn your right palm up and, keeping your arm in contact with the floor, raise your arm up toward your right ear. Stay here for a few breaths, focusing on where your body is supported by the earth beneath you and relaxing into that support. With each exhale silently repeat the mantra *Vam*. Repeat on the other side.

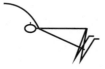

Supine Twist

10. Knees-to-Chest Pose (*Apanasana*)

Hug the knees into the chest. Rest here for a few breaths. Silently repeat the affirmation 3 times: *I trust myself. My inner wisdom guides me.*

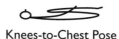

Knees-to-Chest Pose

11. Short relaxation or Sacral Chakra Meditation

You can either finish your practice with a few minutes lying down in the Relaxation Pose (*Savasana*) or, if you have time, find a comfortable seated position and do the Sacral Chakra Meditation that follows the overview of this practice.

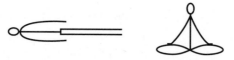

Short relaxation or Sacral Chakra Meditation

Sacral Chakra Yoga Practice Overview

1. Sacral Chakra Awareness Exercise

2. Pelvic rocking. Inhale: *I trust myself.* Exhale: *My inner wisdom guides me.*

3. Pelvic rocking and arm movements × 6

4. Supine Twist and mantra *Vam* × 6 each side

5. Bridge Pose into Knees-to-Chest Pose × 4–6

6. Kneeling *Vam* Sequence × 4–6

7. Seated Twist variation and mantra *Vam*

8. Seated Forward Bend × 6. Inhale: *I trust myself.* Exhale: *My inner wisdom guides me.*

9. Supine Twist and mantra *Vam*

10. Knees-to-Chest Pose. Silently affirm × 3, *I trust myself. My inner wisdom guides me.*

11. Short relaxation or Sacral Chakra Meditation

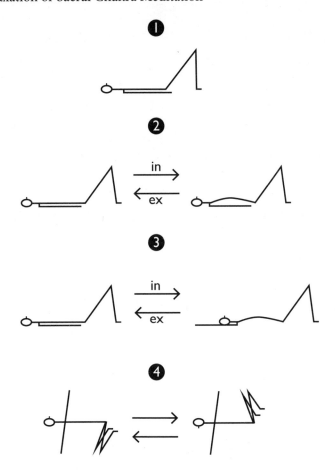

Sacral Chakra Yoga Practice Overview

5

6

7 **8**

9 **10**

11

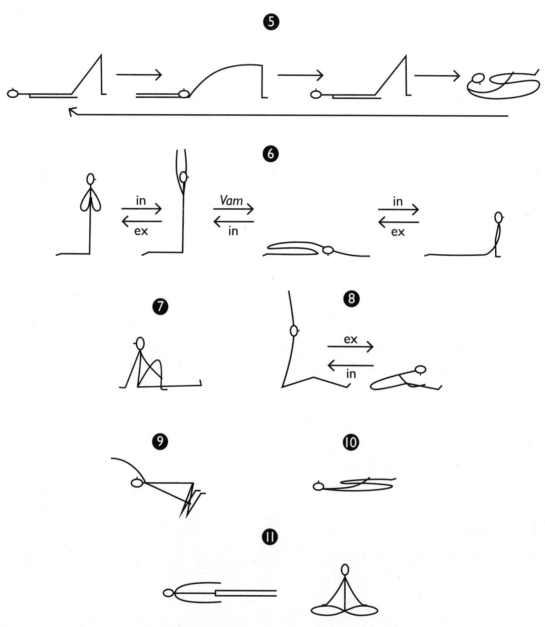

Sacral Chakra Yoga Practice Overview (continued)

MEDITATION

Sacral Chakra Meditation

This meditation can be used to begin or end a yoga practice, but it can also be used on its own as a standalone practice.

Use this meditation anytime you feel uncentered or uncertain about which path to take in life. This meditation is centering and will help you to connect with your intuition and inner wisdom.

Find yourself a comfortable position, either seated or lying. Now bring your awareness to the lower abdomen, the area between the top of the pubic bone and the navel, which is the part of the body associated with the sacral chakra.

Keep your awareness in the belly and silently repeat the chakra's affirmation several times, coordinating it with the breath:

Inhale: I trust myself.

Exhale: My inner wisdom guides me.

Then, let go of the affirmation and, keeping your awareness in the belly, visualize an orange flower. Picture the color and shape of the flower. Notice whether it is open or in bud.

Now let go of picturing the flower and bring your awareness to the natural ebb and flow of the breath. Notice how the belly gently rises and falls with each breath cycle. Notice how there is a wavelike quality to the breath. Each time you exhale, gently contract the lower abdomen, and silently say the mantra *Vam* (pronounced *vum*). Each time you inhale, relax the belly and let the in-breath happen. If you are in a seated position, chant the *Vam* mantra aloud several times.

When you are ready, let go of the chanting. Enjoy the silence. Then notice where your body is in contact with the floor or your support. Take this centered feeling into the next activity you do today.

MEDITATION

Sacral Chakra Walking Meditation

This is a centering meditation. It encourages a positive mindset, it is calming, it shifts rigidity of mind, and it encourages a sense of flow. In the meditation we center ourselves, we are aware of the flow of the breath as we walk, and we're on the lookout for beauty and anything that brings us pleasure. Ideally the walk is done outside.

Begin the meditation by simply being aware of how it feels to be someone walking. With every step notice the sensations associated with your feet making contact with the earth beneath you. Be aware of the rhythm of your walking, noticing how it feels to walk slowly and how it feels to increase the pace. Then drop your awareness down to your lower belly, maintain that centered awareness as you walk, and at the same time, be aware of the natural ebb and flow of your breath.

The human mind is hardwired to notice the negative. However, if you only notice what is wrong as you walk, then it will bring you down. So in this walking meditation make a conscious effort to notice what is beautiful and brings you pleasure—a flower in bud, the color of autumn leaves, a child's smile, a mischievous puppy, or the sun dancing upon water.

When you have finished the walking meditation, resolve to take this positive, centered attitude into the next activity you do today.

MEDITATION
Sacral Chakra Writing Meditation

For full instructions on how to do a writing meditation go to the Writing Meditation with Focus section (see page 44).

Set your timer for 10 to 20 minutes and write meditatively on one of the following subjects:

- Water
- Orange
- Sensual pleasures
- The ebb and flow of life
- My creativity is nurtured by ...

If writing isn't your thing, feel free to work with the above topics in any other medium. For example, paint a picture, make a collage, compose a song, or take some photos, working with the above themes.

Sacral Chakra Meditation Questions

For full instructions on how to use the meditation questions, see page 47.

- When my creativity is blocked, what gets it flowing again?
- What brings me pleasure?
- How easy do I find it to state my preferences?
- Am I in touch with my emotions and able to express how I feel?
- How developed is my intuition and do I attend to the messages I receive from my inner wisdom?

CHAPTER 7

Solar Plexus Chakra (Manipura)

Empower Your Creativity

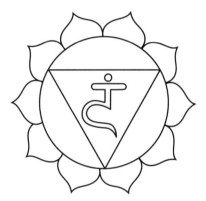

Solar Plexus Chakra Symbol

This chakra empowers you to radiate your creative light out into the world. It gives you the confidence to shine! Working with this chakra helps you develop an ability to take up creative space in the world. It fires up your creativity, and you find the will, the push, and the drive to get your creations out into the world.

The Solar Plexus Chakra at a Glance

Sanskrit Name: *Manipura* (lustrous gem)

Physical Location: Between navel and base of sternum

Element: Fire

Color: Yellow

Yantra: Upward-pointing triangle

Seed Mantra: Ram (pronounced *rum*)

Affirmations: *My inner sun empowers me. I radiate love and light.*

Main Creative Concerns: Firing up creativity and building the confidence to get your creations out into the world.

Balanced: Self-aware, self-assured, self-confident, assertive, expressive, takes up space, stands their ground, bold, channels anger into creating change, courageous, sunny, optimistic, radiates light out into the world.

Excessive: Domineering, overconfident, bullying, disrespectful of others' space, reckless, expresses anger destructively, poor self-awareness, blocks out the sun for others.

Deficient: Shrinking violet, lack of confidence, fearful, reserved, easily swayed, pushover, timid, repressed, pushes down anger, stands in the shadow.

Life Issues: Self-empowerment, developing a sense of self, assertiveness, right to take up space, building self-confidence, overcoming challenges, finding your place in the world; building physical, mental, and emotional strength.

Healing Practices: Strength-training exercises, boxing yoga, martial arts, power walking, running, assertiveness training, anger management, sunny days, psychic protection, acquiring skills and increasing confidence, taking calculated risks, positive self-talk.

Solar-Powered Creativity!

The first chakra is concerned with our tribal identity, the second chakra revolves around forming relationships, and the third chakra enables us to form a sense of personal identity. The work we have done on the two lower chakras will support us in our quest to discover who we are and to express ourselves through our creativity. Our work with the solar plexus chakra is to locate the sun at our center and to shine that light out into the world. Yoga helps you stand tall and find the courage in your heart to follow your true creative path in life.

Yoga, like many spiritual and religious traditions, emphasizes the need to let go of the ego in order to become enlightened. However, one must first have developed an ego, or a sense of self, in order to transcend it. To be a creative force in the world, you do need a strong sense of self. It takes courage and a strong dose of self-belief to raise your head above the parapet and push your creations out into the world for all to see. Whether you are exhibiting a picture, publishing a novel, erecting a statue, blogging, or even tweeting, it can be both exhilarating and terrifying. What if people hate it? What if I make a fool of myself? What if I am rejected? Working on the first two chakras helps build a stable, supportive base for our creativity, and now the third chakra helps us build the self-confidence, strength, and resilience that we need to see any creative project through to completion.

There's a phenomenal amount of work to be done before you get to the point of having an art exhibition, publishing a book, releasing a movie, and the like. You must have the self-confidence to fight for your entitlement to take the time, space, and resources that you need to manifest your creative vision. Women are often raised to be selfless, and they must develop the ego in order to stake out their creative territory and overcome their conditioning of always putting other peoples' needs before their own. Your vision is unique; it would be such a loss to the world if through fear of being selfish your words go unwritten, unread, or your insightful wisdom goes unexpressed and is forever lost. Turn it around: it's not selfish to write—it's selfish not to share your creative gifts with the world! Yes, the arts can be perceived of as self-indulgent. However, without artists' contribution, the world would be an impoverished and monochrome place.

Working on the third chakra is empowering. The sort of power we are referring to is not "power over." Rather, it is the power to locate the sun at your center and shine that light into the world. In this way you will become a beacon and light the way for others. We need writers, painters, and other creative visionaries to illuminate a fresh way of viewing the world and inspire us all to work for change.

Creativity helps us to break free from the wheel of habitual behavior, to step out of the norm, and to try something new. This might sometimes ruffle feathers, so as artists we need to have a strong sense of self, cultivated through our work on the third chakra, to weather the storm of public opinion, a bad review, or disapproval. It's an act of generosity to share your creations with the world. It's also a risky business. You might be applauded for your efforts, but there is always a chance that you will be ridiculed and shamed. In the latter case, the work you do on the third chakra will help you pick yourself up, dust yourself off, and try again.

What is it that prevents us from shining our light out into the world? Artists have a reputation for being unconventional, mavericks who flout society's rules. This is seen as admirable in men and shocking in women. Social norms restrict women's expression, and to be an artist and a woman is an act of subversion. When women raise their heads above the parapet and express themselves, they are often silenced by being shamed about their appearance. Women are frequently shamed and intimidated on social media. Many women do stand up to this and still tweet, blog, and get their vision out into the world. Working on the third chakra will empower you to keep on keeping on and to maintain a sense of self-belief whatever the world throws at you. Nevertheless, she persisted!

The third chakra houses the fiery energy of anger. In some spiritual circles anger is viewed as a "negative" emotion that is to be eradicated. I find this view disempowering. When we feel anger, this powerful emotion is signaling to us that our boundaries have been breached and we need to do something to protect ourselves. We ignore anger at our peril. When we repress anger, it turns in upon us and can lead to depression. However, if we simply act out our angry impulses, it is likely that someone will get hurt and we will end up regretting it. An alternative is to quieten down and listen to your anger. What is it trying to tell you? What needs to change? Suppressed anger can stifle creativity, whereas righteous anger, when mindfully acted upon, can turbocharge creativity and be a force for radical change.

Remember to be on the lookout for role models, those individuals who are beacons, demonstrating to us that despite facing incredible obstacles in their lives, they still shine brightly and light the way for the rest of us.

Commitment Empowers Creativity

Some of you reading this book will be turning to creative activities to enhance your well-being and to relieve stress. Perhaps it's something you do in your spare time to create balance in a busy life. However, others of you might wish to deepen your practice of creativity and to take it to another level. Either way this section will give you some tips and suggestions that will help you to deepen your creative practice. If you find it difficult to see a project through, then read on. This section is for you.

Take a moment to consider: What does the word *commitment* conjure up for you? Is there a heaviness about the word that turns you off? When you first set out on the creative path, just as when you first start dating, it can be good to try out lots of different things and discover what turns you on and makes you feel fully alive. Like a bee flying from flower to flower, you can try out lots of creative pursuits, activities, techniques, methods, and approaches. However, at some point, once you know what's on offer, it is beneficial to commit to a particular discipline and deepen your understanding of it. If the idea of commitment sounds a bit heavy for you, no worries. Start by just dipping your toe in the water, and then decide later whether you want to take the plunge and dive in.

When a person flits from relationship to relationship, they might be referred to as "commitment-phobic." Of course, when we first start dating, it can be fun to play the field, but when the magic and romance of starting a relationship fades, it can be tempting to move on to get back the thrill of first love. However, if we always give up at the first sign of difficulty in a relationship, we miss out on the depth of love and experience that comes from committing to and working through difficulties. Likewise, if we wish to deepen our relationship with creativity, then commitment is an essential ingredient.

Instead of talking about commitment, it might be helpful to reframe it and instead think about setting an intention, which is a great way to power up your creativity. Initially, you might simply set an intention to commit to spending a certain amount of time each day doing a creative activity. Even five minutes a day can have a beneficial effect and get your creative juices flowing. Remember you're more likely to stick to this gentle discipline and apply yourself if you choose an activity that you enjoy doing. The seeds of creativity can be planted in many ways; for you it might be spending five minutes doing mindful coloring, creative baking, reading a book, trying out a new yoga sequence, journaling, or whatever else appeals to you.

Many of us have internalized the cliché that you must suffer for your art. However, if your art is more about suffering than enjoyment, then it's worth considering whether you're on the wrong path. Naturally, not every aspect of the creative process will be enjoyable, and on any creative journey there will be highs and lows. Commitment is about sticking with the process and wading through the swamp because you want to see the stunning views from the top of the mountain.

Commitment helps you see a project through. For example, imagine you are knitting a jumper and then you get to a fiddly bit that requires shaping. This turns out to be more difficult than you first thought, and you feel like giving up. You can choose to put away the knitting and forget about it—maybe knitting isn't for you—or you can go online and watch a YouTube video on how to shape a jumper and persevere until you are the proud wearer of a beautiful, unique hand-knitted jumper. If you choose the latter, it will build your confidence, improve your skills, and empower you to try new ventures. The same principle applies to bigger projects, such as writing a novel, painting a full-size canvas, and composing a symphony; committing to the project and being prepared to work through the difficulties yields wonderful results and along the way will help you to grow and develop as a person.

When you set your intention and commit to a project, you create the right conditions for miracles to happen! As the mountaineer William Hutchison Murray wrote, "The moment one definitely commits oneself, then Providence moves too. All sorts of things occur to help one that would never otherwise have occurred. A whole stream of events issues from the decision, raising in one's favour all manner of unforeseen incidents and meetings and material assistance, which no man could have dreamt would have come his way."[28]

So when we work with the third chakra, we discover that willpower, determination, strength, and persistence are all our allies in the creative process. However, please note that brute force and grim determination are not. The muse does not respond well to being bullied into performing, and she is much more likely to reward you with a brilliant idea if you coax her with the power of kindness. Creativity serves us best when we slow back down to body speed, rather than racing ahead of ourselves and trying to keep up with mind speed. If you find yourself trying too hard, getting impatient, and failing to push ideas out, then stop, pause, take a break, go for a walk, meet up with a friend, and come back later refreshed and ready to go again. Your other option, for those times when you find yourself slipping into grim determination mode, is to either slip down a gear to the sacral chakra and get back into your flow, or slip up a gear to the heart chakra and give yourself and the creative process some loving kindness.

Yoga Inspired by the Solar Plexus Chakra

This chakra is ruled by the sun and its element is fire. We can use sun imagery to bring a fiery, uplifting quality to a solar plexus chakra–inspired yoga practice. During the practice, we visualize a warm, glowing sun at the solar plexus and picture sunlight radiating

---

28. William Hutchison Murray, *The Scottish Himalayan Expedition* (London: J. M. Dent & Sons, 1951), 6–7

warmth and light out from our center and around the body. We are aiming to find the sun at the center of our life and to shine that light out into the world.

This chakra is concerned with confidence building and assertiveness, and so we choose expansive poses that encourage us to take up space, such as all versions of the Warrior Pose (*Virabhadrasana*) and Triangle Pose (*Trikonasana*), and combine them with sun imagery creating a sense of radiating in the poses. We also use strengthening poses such as Chair Pose (*Utkatasana*) or Plank Pose (*Chaturanga Dandasana*).

The empowering seed mantra *Ram* (pronounced *rum*), associated with this chakra, can be used as part of a meditation or combined with dynamic yoga movements. We temper the fiery quality of the solar plexus chakra by including the compassionate seed mantra *Yam*, associated with the heart chakra (*anahata*). Stability is created and our connection to the earth strengthened by chanting the seed mantra *Lam*, which is associated with the earthy root chakra (*muladhara*).

Yellow is the color associated with this chakra, and we introduce a warm, sunny optimism into the practice by visualizing a yellow flower at the solar plexus center.

Solar Plexus Chakra Yoga Practice

You can use this sunny practice anytime you want to build up confidence, courage, and inner strength. It will connect you to your fiery, assertive self, while at the same time helping you get in touch with your loving heart. It is energizing, revitalizing, and grounding and creates stability. It's the go-to yoga practice whenever you need to be nurtured and empowered.

The affirmations we use in the practice are *My inner sun empowers me* and *I radiate love and light*. They can be coordinated with the breath:

Inhale: My inner sun empowers me.

Exhale: I radiate love and light.

Allow 20 to 30 minutes.

At the end of these instructions, you'll find an illustrated aide-mémoire for the whole practice.

1. Solar Plexus Chakra Awareness Exercise, seated

Find yourself a comfortable sitting position. Now bring your awareness to the solar plexus (the area below your breastbone but above your navel). Keep your awareness at the solar plexus and silently repeat the chakra's affirmation several times, coordinating it with the breath. Inhale and affirm, *My inner sun empowers me.* Exhale and affirm, *I radiate love and light.*

Then, let go of the affirmation and picture a sun radiating warmth, light, and energy at your solar plexus.

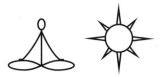

Solar Plexus Chakra Awareness Exercise, seated

2. Mountain Pose (*Tadasana*) with sun visualization

Stand in Mountain Pose (*Tadasana*). In your mind's eye visualize the sun in the sky. Now picture a warm, glowing sun at your solar plexus, radiating warmth and light.

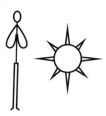

Mountain Pose with sun visualization

3. Warrior 1 (*Virabhadrasana* 1) variation

Stand tall, feet hip width apart, turn your left foot slightly out, and take a big step forward with your right leg. Place your hands on your solar plexus. Inhaling, bend your right knee, opening your arms out wide to the side. Exhaling, straighten your right leg and bring your hands back to your solar plexus. You can coordinate the breath with the affirmation. Inhale and affirm, *My inner sun empowers me.* Exhale and affirm, *I radiate love and light.* Do 6 repetitions on this side and then repeat on the other side.

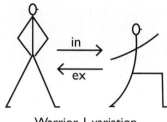

Warrior I variation

4. Warrior 1 (*Virabhadrasana* 1) with sun visualization

Stand tall, feet hip width apart, turn your left foot slightly out, and take a big step forward with your right leg. Take both arms overhead, bringing the palms of the hands together (for a gentler pose have the hands shoulder width apart). Picture a warm, glowing sun at your solar plexus, radiating warmth and light. Stay for a few breaths. Repeat on the other side.

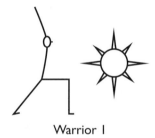

Warrior I

5. *Ram-Yam-Lam* Sequence

Stand tall, feet parallel and about hip width apart, with hands resting on the solar plexus. Inhale and take the arms out to the sides. On the exhale, chant *Ram* (pronounced *rum*), as you bring your hands back to the solar plexus. Inhale taking the arms overhead. Exhale, lowering the arms and crossing the hands to the heart, as you chant *Yam* (pronounced *yum*). Inhale, taking the arms overhead. Exhale, coming into a Standing Forward Bend (*Uttanasana*), chanting *Lam* (pronounced *lum*). Inhale, come back up to standing, taking both arms up above the head. Exhale, lowering the hands back to the solar plexus. Repeat the sequence 3 more times.

If you are short of time, you can end your practice here.

Ram-Yam-Lam Sequence

6. Strengthening Salute to the Sun (*Surya Namaskar* variation)

Repeat 2 to 4 rounds of the following sequence:

6a. Mountain Pose (*Tadasana*) with sun visualization

Stand in Mountain Pose (*Tadasana*) with your hands in Prayer Position (*Namaste*). In your mind's eye visualize the sun in the sky. Now picture a warm, glowing sun at your solar plexus, radiating warmth and light, and keep this image in mind as you perform the Salute to the Sun (*Surya Namaskar*) variation.

Mountain Pose

6b. Chair Pose (*Utkatasana*)

Stand tall, feet hip width apart and both arms above your head. Bend your knees and lower your bottom as if to sit down on a high stool. Keep the ears between the arms and don't round the upper back. Imagine that your hips are being pulled downward and everything above the waist is reaching skyward. Stay for a few breaths.

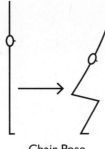

Chair Pose

6c. Standing Forward Bend (*Uttanasana*)

From Chair Pose (*Utkatasana*) allow your body to melt down into a Standing Forward Bend (*Uttanasana*). Then bend the knees and arch the back, and come back down into the forward bend.

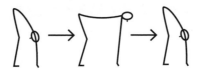

Standing Forward Bend

6d. Plank Pose (*Chaturanga Dandasana*)

Step the legs back, one at a time, into Plank Pose (*Chaturanga Dandasana*), holding the whole body in one long line.

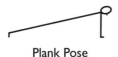

Plank Pose

6e. Plank Pose (*Chaturanga Dandasana*) into Half Press-Ups

From Plank Pose (*Chaturanga Dandasana*) lower the knees to the floor into a half press-up position. Do 4 press-ups, keeping the head, torso, and thighs in one long line. (For a stronger version keep the legs straight and do full press-ups.)

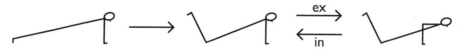

Plank Pose into Half Press-Ups

6f. Plank Pose (*Chaturanga Dandasana*) into Child's Pose (*Balasana*)

From Plank Pose (*Chaturanga Dandasana*) drop the knees to the floor, sitting back into Child's Pose (*Balasana*), and rest here for a few breaths.

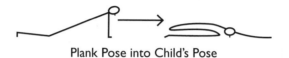

Plank Pose into Child's Pose

6g. Child's Pose (*Balasana*) into Upward-Facing Dog Pose (*Urdhva Mukha Svanasana*)

From Child's Pose (*Balasana*) come into Upward-Facing Dog Pose (*Urdhva Mukha Svanasana*).

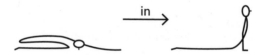

Child's Pose into Upward-Facing Dog Pose

6h. Downward-Facing Dog Pose (*Adho Mukha Svanasana*)

From Upward-Facing Dog Pose (*Urdhva Mukha Svanasana*) turn the toes under and swing back into a Downward-Facing Dog Pose (*Adho Mukha Svanasana*). Stay for a few breaths in the pose.

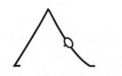

Downward-Facing Dog Pose

6i. Lunge Pose (*Anjaneyasana*)

From Downward-Facing Dog Pose (*Adho Mukha Svanasana*) bring your right foot forward into Lunge Pose (*Anjaneyasana*).

Lunge Pose

6j. Standing Forward Bend (*Uttanasana*)

Bring the back foot forward, coming into a Standing Forward Bend (*Uttanasana*). Bend the knees and arch the back. Come back into the Standing Forward Bend and stay for a few breaths.

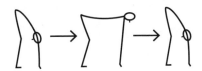

Standing Forward Bend

6k. Mountain Pose (*Tadasana*) with sun visualization

From the Forward Bend, sweep the arms out to the sides and up above the head, coming back up to standing. Lower the hands back into the Prayer Position (*Namaste*) and rest here for a few breaths. As you rest, picture a warm, glowing sun at your solar plexus, radiating warmth and light, and keep this image in mind as you perform another round of the Salute to the Sun. Do between 2 and 4 rounds.

Finish here or move on to step 7.

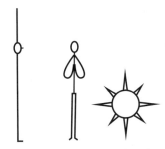

Mountain Pose with sun visualization

7. Seated Forward Bend (*Paschimottanasana*) and mantra *Ram*

Sit tall with legs outstretched (bend the knees to ease the pose). Bring your awareness to the solar plexus. Picture a warm, radiant sun there. Inhale and raise arms. Keeping your awareness at the solar plexus, exhale and chant the mantra *Ram* (pronounced *rum*). At the end of the exhale, as you complete the chant, fold forward over the legs. Inhale and return to starting position. Repeat 6 times, and on the final time stay for a few breaths in the Seated Forward Bend. Note: never strain with the breathing. Take extra breaths if you need to.

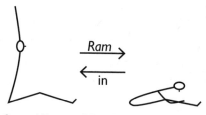

Seated Forward Bend and mantra *Ram*

8. Heart Chakra Sequence

Start in Child's Pose (*Balasana*), with forearms and hands on the floor, just above your head. Inhale and come up to tall kneeling, taking your arms above your head. Exhale, chanting the mantra *Yam* (pronounced *yum*), as you cross your hands and place them at your heart. Inhale, raising the arms above your head again. Exhale, coming back to Child's Pose. Repeat the sequence 6 times.

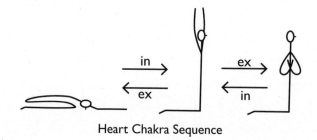

Heart Chakra Sequence

9. Short relaxation or Solar Plexus Chakra Meditation

Either finish your practice here with a short relaxation in the Relaxation Pose (*Savasana*) or come to sitting and do the Solar Plexus Chakra Meditation that follows.

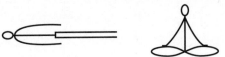

Short Relaxation or Solar Plexus Chakra Meditation

Solar Plexus Chakra Yoga Practice Overview

1. Solar Plexus Chakra Awareness Exercise

2. Mountain Pose with sun visualization

3. Warrior 1 variation × 6. Inhale: *My inner sun empowers me.* Exhale: *I radiate love and light.* Repeat on other side.

4. Warrior 1 with sun visualization

5. *Ram-Yam-Lam* Sequence × 4. *End here if short of time.*

6. Strengthening Salute to the Sun × 2–4 rounds. *Finish here or move on to step 7.*

7. Seated Forward Bend and mantra *Ram* × 6

8. Heart Chakra Sequence × 6

9. Short relaxation or Solar Plexus Chakra Meditation

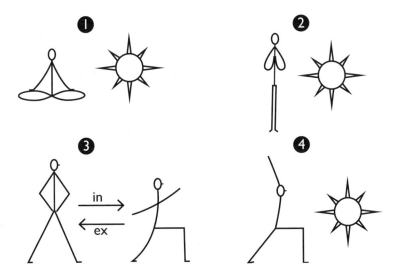

Solar Plexus Chakra Yoga Practice Overview

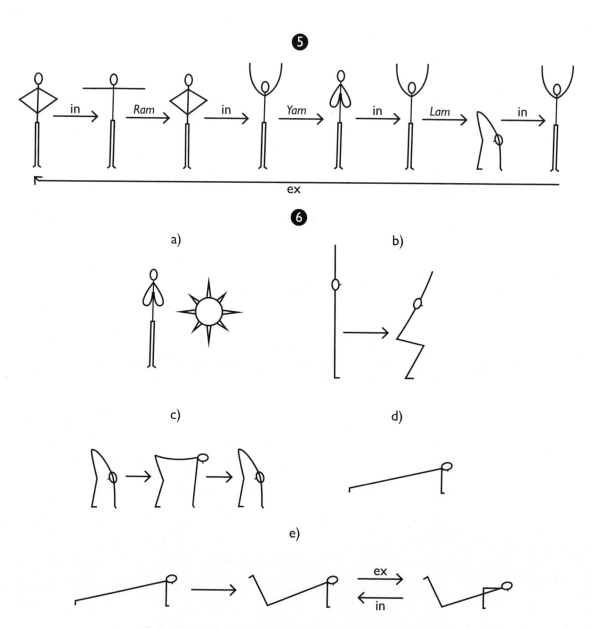

Solar Plexus Chakra Yoga Practice Overview (continued)

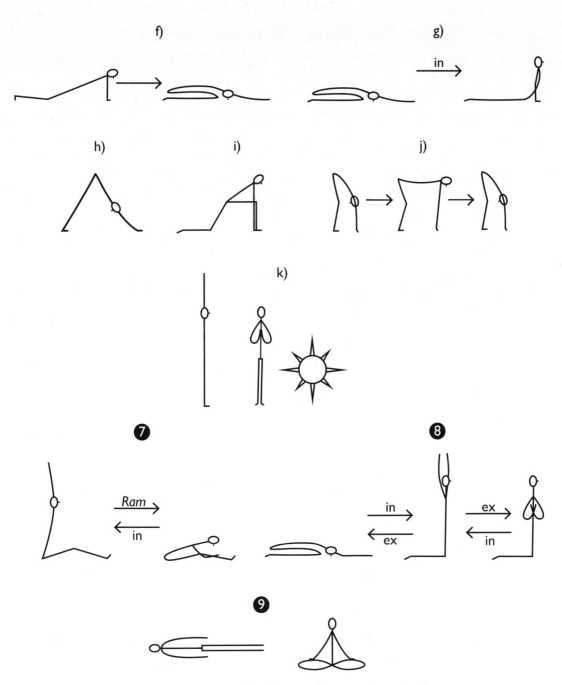

Solar Plexus Chakra Yoga Practice Overview (continued)

Solar Plexus Chakra Meditation

This meditation can be used at the start or finish of a yoga session, and it can also be used on its own as a standalone practice.

You can use this sunny meditation anytime you feel that a cloud is hanging over you, and its sunny energy will disperse the storm clouds and leave you feeling stronger and happier. It is energizing, revitalizing, uplifting, and empowering.

Find yourself a comfortable position, either sitting or lying down. Now bring your awareness to the solar plexus (the area below your breastbone but above your navel), which is the part of the body associated with this chakra.

Keep your awareness at the solar plexus and visualize a yellow flower. Picture the color and shape of the flower. Notice whether it is open or in bud. Enjoy the beauty of the flower.

Now let go of picturing the flower and keeping your awareness at the solar plexus, silently repeat the affirmation for the practice several times, coordinating it with the breath:

Inhale: My inner sun empowers me.

Exhale: I radiate love and light.

Then, let go of the affirmation and picture a sun radiating warmth, light, and energy at your solar plexus. Imagine that as you inhale you are breathing into the sun at your solar plexus, and as you exhale you are breathing out from there. Repeat for a few breaths. Now imagine that with each inhale the sun is charged up, and on each exhale the sun expands and glows a little brighter.

Inhale: Charge up

Exhale: Expand

After a few breaths of breathing in this way, begin to send the sun's healing rays all around your body. With each inhale the sun is recharged, and with each exhale the sun is radiating healing rays of light all around the body.

Inhale: Recharge

Exhale: Radiate

Now let go of the image of the sun but keep your awareness resting in the solar plexus area. Inhale, and on the exhale silently repeat the mantra *Ram* (pronounced *rum*). Repeat several times. And then, if you are sitting, repeat the mantra aloud several times.

When you are ready, let go of chanting the mantra. Enjoy the silence. Resolve to take this sunny, empowered attitude into the next thing you do today.

EXERCISE

Solar Plexus Chakra Solar-Powered Walking Meditation

You can do this walking meditation anytime you need to boost your confidence or uplift your mood. Ideally, walk outside in the fresh air.

At the start of your walk, think about your posture. Stand tall, head held high, shoulders back and down. Ask yourself the question, "How would I walk if I were a super confident person?" And then walk in that super confident way!

Picture a warm, glowing sun at your solar plexus radiating warmth and light, and keep this image in mind as you walk. Whereas generally we slow the pace down for a walking meditation, for this one we walk briskly. If you pass by another walker, if it feels right to do so, smile and say hello. Share your warm sunny attitude with them!

If it's a sunny day, be aware of the warmth of the sun on your skin or sunlight dancing on water. Notice sunlight and shadow. If it isn't sunny, remind yourself that the sun is still there behind the clouds.

If you have been walking at a brisk pace, gradually slow your pace down to your usual walking pace. Resolve to take this sunny, confident attitude into the rest of your day.

MEDITATION

Solar Plexus Chakra Writing Meditation

For full instructions on how to do a writing meditation, go to the Writing Meditation with Focus section (see page 44).

Set your timer for 10 to 20 minutes and write meditatively on one of the following subjects:

- Fire
- Power
- The sun
- Yellow
- Assertiveness

If writing isn't your thing, feel free to work with the above topics in any other medium. For example, paint a picture, make a collage, compose a song, or take some photos, working with the above themes.

Solar Plexus Chakra Meditation Questions

For full instructions on how to use the meditation questions, see page 47.

- What fires up my creativity?
- Am I able to defend my creative need for time, space, and resources?
- Who are the beacons who inspire my creativity?
- How resilient am I when dealing with criticism of my work?
- What would I need to do to cultivate unshakeable self-confidence and self-belief?

CHAPTER 8

Heart Chakra
(Anahata)

Locate the Loving Heart at the Center of Creativity

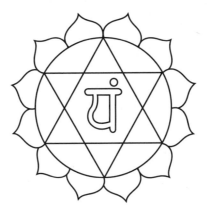

Heart Chakra Symbol

This chakra breathes life and love into your creations. It helps you find a point of balance between heaven and earth, resulting in your creations being harmonious and balanced. Working with this chakra teaches you to show compassion and love to yourself and others as you tread the creative path.

The Heart Chakra at a Glance

Sanskrit Name: *Anahata* (wheel of the unstruck sound)

Physical Location: Center of the chest, lungs, heart circulatory system

Element: Air

Colors: Pink, green

Yantra: Hexagon

Seed Mantra: *Yam* (pronounced *yum*)

Affirmations: *My spacious heart holds all. My loving heart heals all.*

Main Creative Concern: Being guided by the heart to create transformative, soulful work that unites the material and spiritual, bringing peace and healing.

Balanced: Strikes a healthy balance between giving and receiving love, compassionate toward self and others, empathy, in touch with emotions, heart and head work together, good work-life balance, sense of fair play, calls out injustice, altruistic, balances doing with simply being.

Excessive: Needy, looks to others for fulfillment and completion, codependency, addictive, lack of self-esteem, fails to set boundaries, sentimental, overconcern with romantic love, idealist.

Deficient: Defensive, aloof, lonely, fearful of getting hurt, tight, tense, contracted, cynical, disillusioned, not able to give or receive love.

Life Issues: Forming loving, healthy relationships, uniting the spiritual and the material, finding equilibrium, establishing healthy rhythms that balance work and play, creating a fair and just world.

Healing Practices: Relaxation, meditation, mindful self-compassion, mindfulness, pranayama, cardiovascular exercise, laughter, seeking out beauty, being in nature, awareness of biorhythms, awareness of nature's seasonal cycles, observing lunar cycles, giving and receiving love, random acts of kindness, working for peace and justice, connecting with any form of art, literature, or music that speaks to your soul.

Find Your Creative Pulse

At the center of all our lives is the dance of the beating heart. Creativity, like the heartbeat, has a rhythm and pulse: it alternates between periods of doing and times of simply being.

Society favors relentless activity, so it is going against the grain to stop and simply be. However, manic activity doesn't always produce the best work. Like many writers, I often find my best ideas come at those in-between times, when I'm walking, in the shower, or doing a mundane household task.

Everything moves in cycles. Earth spins around the sun, night follows day, the seasons turn—spring, summer, autumn, winter, and then spring comes around again. The dance of life, the pulse of life. Nature's way is for periods of activity to be followed by periods of rest. Relentless activity wears down the creative impulse. It is important to follow periods of intense activity with a period of rest. We empty ourselves in order to create the space to receive again. Creative inspiration cannot be forced; it is a state of grace. You can work to create the right conditions for inspiration to arise, but sometimes it's a question of waiting patiently, listening, and allowing yourself to be filled up.

Creativity likes to flow. A constricted heart is an obstacle to the free flow of creative energy. Breathe. The natural way of all things is ebb and flow. A pulsing, an expansion, followed by a condensing. Periods of activity followed by periods of rest. Impatience with the creative rhythm can cause us to try to force the process. Sometimes this works and results in a breakthrough. However, to sustain a longtime creative practice it's important to respect the pulse of the creative process. Pushing and yielding.

When we are impatient, our breathing is often shallow and constricted. By attending to the natural flow of the breath, we return to a receptive state where ideas can flow again. Breathe in, pause, breathe out, pause. We do not force the breath; we simply observe that at the end of each in-breath, before we breathe out, there is a natural pause. And at the end of each out-breath, before we breathe in, there is a natural pause. The pause is a spacious place where we rest and wait, trusting in the process of breathing. Breathing in, we expand and take in life energy. Breathing out, we let go and relax. At the end of the exhale, we wait, we pause, we relax, and we let the in-breath fill us up, inspire us. We are literally inspired!

The lungs are like balloons. They fill with air, then like bellows they empty. The pulse of life, alternating between empty and full. Giving and receiving. The pregnant pause. Listen to your heart, let it guide you on your way, and your path will be a heartfelt one.

What is your creative rhythm? What is the pulse at the heart of your creative practice? The heart chakra seeks equilibrium, homeostasis, and balance. Remember to feed your creativity by taking in nourishment from the world around you, and then give back to the world the gift of your lovingly made creations. By pausing and waiting to be filled up, you clear the way for divine energy to be channeled through you. Listen, listen to your beating heart. Seek and find passion, union, relationship, and compassion. Give and take. Allow yourself to be filled up, to receive grace.

Locating the Beating Heart of Your Creativity

What is the beating heart at the center of your creativity? What motivates you to spend hours, days, months, and even years on your creative endeavors? What do you love? What is your passion? What is it that breathes life into your creations?

The heart is the moderator, circulating ideas and pumping lifeblood into your creations. As a creative person, are you looking after yourself? Are you balancing and attending to your physical, mental, emotional, and spiritual needs? Looking after yourself is like feeding the soil in your garden so healthy plants can grow.

Kintsugi is the Japanese art of repairing broken pottery with glue dusted with powdered gold, highlighting the cracks and repairs. In this way that which was broken is celebrated as an object of beauty. Compassion for ourselves and others arises in our heart when life is lived through us, and it is the gold dust in the glue, bringing humanity to our creations. When the heart is at the center of our creativity, then our work is grounded in material reality and elevated to spiritual heights. The heart heals the rift between lower and higher, material and spiritual, earth and heaven. Where the heart finds fragmentation and brokenness, it glues the disparate parts back together, illuminating the scarred join with gold dust. What is broken is healed and made whole by our heartfelt creative endeavors.

Creativity is passion, love, and healing. In order for your creativity to be heartfelt, it must come from a place of love. This is not a sentimental love, it is bold and courageous, a fighting force for justice, peace, equality, and a fairer world. At the same time creativity is often surreal, irrational, amoral, and an expression of a deeper source of wisdom. Our ability to show love and compassion toward ourselves and others is as much a marker of success as our outer achievements. The heart chakra is the door to love and relationships. Let us create in a heartfelt way.

The loving heart holds our anger, our fear, and our doubt. At the same time it reminds us of what has been lost, what is beautiful and good, and it shows us a world that is worth fighting for. Our work may have begun as a catalog of all that is wrong in the world, but we look to the heart to remind us that the forces of love are stronger than the forces of hate. Love sustains our efforts, love holds our hurt, love provides us with a healing balm.

Creativity needs spaciousness and room to breathe. Creativity that arises from a loving heart is sustainable and can still be cutting edge, challenging, and subversive. We are right to be angry about injustice. We are right to channel our creativity to bring about change, but we do not want the forces of hatred to score a victory over our heart. A loving heart sees all the woe in the world but at the same time has a vision of what a just, fair world could look like. Justice or just is? Creativity is a force for change. The heart balances all.

Yoga Inspired by the Heart Chakra

The heart chakra mediates between the world of matter and spirit, creating an energetic, figure eight-like pathway flowing between the lower, foundational chakras, and the higher, celestial ones. The three "lower" chakras below the heart are associated with material, earthly concerns, and the three "higher" chakras above the heart are associated with more spiritual matters.

When working with the heart chakra, it's important to maintain an awareness of the chakras above and the chakras below the heart. Be aware of where your body is in contact with the earth and relax into that support, while simultaneously noticing the space around your body and feeling yourself expanding into that space. The *Chandogya Upanishad* states that "the little space within the heart is as great as this vast universe. The heavens and the earth are there, and the sun, and the moon, and the stars … the whole universe … dwells within our heart."[29]

The elements associated with the previous chakras were earth, water, and fire, and now with the heart chakra we move into the intangibility of air. Above all, with this chakra we are aware of the breath, as the breath is the umbilical cord that connects us to life itself. In the heart chakra yoga practice that follows we use the breathing to engender a sense of spaciousness and freedom. We also connect with beauty and a sense of the heart blossoming by visualizing a pink lotus flower on a bed of green leaves. Pink and green are the colors associated with the heart chakra.

The chakras below the heart are concerned with tribal love, sexual love, and self-love, whereas the heart chakra is associated with unconditional love. In our yoga practice when working with the heart chakra we choose heart-opening poses such as Cobra Pose

---

29. Mascaro, trans., *The Upanishads*, 120.

(*Bhujangasana*), Sphinx Pose (*Salamba Bhujangasana*), and Bow Pose (*Dhanurasana*). We also utilize poses that ground, center, and align the body, in accord with the balancing nature of the heart center.

When we work with the heart center, we open ourselves to the potential of powerful emotional healing. In our practice we cultivate a sense of the heart being capable of holding all our emotions, even those that are most troubling and painful. Our spacious heart holds our hurts, and our loving heart heals them. We can encourage this process by making our inner dialog one of kindness and compassion, talking to ourselves with the same love and understanding that we would show a good friend.

Heart Chakra Yoga Practice

This practice creates a sense of mental and physical equilibrium, gently opening the heart. It creates a sense of spaciousness, opening us up to receiving fresh inspiration. The practice also teaches you the nurturing skill of holding and healing your emotions at the heart center, promoting the process of healing.

The affirmations we use in the practice are *My spacious heart holds all* and *My loving heart heals all.* They can be coordinated with the breath:

Inhale: My spacious heart holds all.

Exhale: My loving heart heals all.

Allow 20 to 30 minutes.

At the end of these instructions, you'll find an illustrated aide-mémoire for the whole practice.

1. Heart Chakra Awareness Exercise

Find yourself a comfortable lying position, making sure that you are symmetrically aligned. Bring your awareness to your heart center, silently repeat the heart chakra affirmation a few times, coordinating it with the breath. Inhale and affirm, *My spacious heart holds all.* Exhale and affirm, *My loving heart heals all.*

Now become aware of the natural flow of your breath, observing the breath without imposing a pattern on it. With each breath notice the belly rising and falling and the chest expanding and condensing. Follow the full length of the in-breath and the full length of the out-breath. If your mind wanders off, just gently bring it back to riding the waves of the breath.

At the end of the next in-breath, observe that there is a pause before you exhale, and at the end of the exhale, notice that there is a pause before you inhale. Simply observe the pause and relax into it. There's no need to force it. Let it be easy and effortless. At the end of each exhale, consciously relax your belly, and allow the inhale to arise out of the pause, with no effort on your part. Create space and be inspired by the breath.

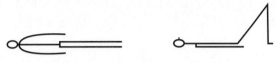

Heart Chakra Awareness Exercise

2. Knees-to-Chest Pose (*Apanasana*) into leg raises

Bring both knees onto your chest. Inhale and straighten your legs vertically, heels toward the ceiling, taking your arms out to the side just below shoulder height, palms facing up. Exhale and bring the knees back to the chest and hands back to the knees. Inhale and affirm, *My spacious heart holds all*. Exhale and affirm, *My loving heart heals all*. Repeat 6 times.

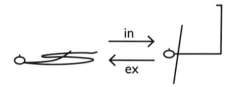

Knees-to-Chest Pose into leg raises

3. Cat Pose (*Marjaryasana*) into Child's Pose (*Balasana*)

Come onto all fours. Exhaling, round the back into Cat Pose and lower the bottom to the heels and the head to the floor into Child's Pose. Pause. Inhaling, come back up to all fours. Pause. As you move, be aware of the natural pause that occurs at the end of the exhalation and the inhalation. Repeat 6 times.

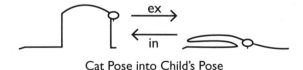

Cat Pose into Child's Pose

4. Mountain Pose (*Tadasana*)

Stand tall, feet parallel and about hip width apart. Be aware of the contact between your feet and the earth beneath you. Imagine a string attached to the crown of your head, gently pulling you skyward; simultaneously, let your tailbone drop and feel your heels rooting down into the earth. Be aware of the space around you. Inhale and affirm, *My spacious heart holds all*. Exhale and affirm, *My loving heart heals all*. Repeat 6 times.

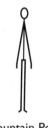

Mountain Pose

5. Warrior 1 (*Virabhadrasana* 1) variation

Stand tall with feet hip width apart, turn your left foot slightly out, and take a big step forward with your right leg, hands crossed at your heart. Inhaling, bend your right knee, opening your arms out wide to the side. Exhaling, chant the mantra *Yam* (pronounced *yum*) as you straighten your right leg and cross your hands at your heart. Inhaling, bend your right knee, this time taking your arms above your head. Exhaling, chant the mantra *Yam* as you straighten your right leg and cross your hands at your heart. Repeat the whole sequence 4 times. Repeat on the other side.

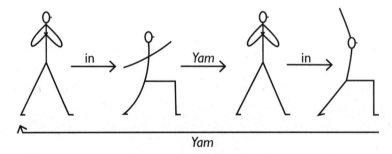

Warrior 1 variation

6. Dancer Pose (*Natarajasana*)

Stand tall, feet hip width apart and arms by your sides. Bend your right knee, and with your right hand catch hold of your ankle. Take the left arm up above the head. Then tip the torso forward, extending the back foot up and away from you and reaching forward and up with the opposite arm. Stay for a few breaths and then repeat on the other side. If you have balance problems, practice facing a wall with your extended hand resting on the wall for support.

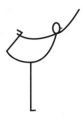

Dancer Pose

7. Floor Salute to the Sun (*Surya Namaskar* variation)

The following are steps for the floor Salute to the Sun (*Surya Namaskar* variation):

7a. Tall kneeling with affirmation

Come to tall kneeling. Cross your hands at your heart silently repeat the affirmation: *My spacious heart holds all. My loving heart heals all.*

Tall kneeling

7b. Tall kneeling into Child's Pose (*Balasana*)

Inhale, raising both arms above your head. Exhale, folding forward into Child's Pose (*Balasana*).

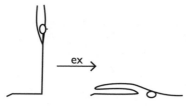

Tall kneeling into Child's Pose

7c. All fours into Downward-Facing Dog Pose (*Adho Mukha Svanasana*)

Inhale, coming onto all fours, and turn the toes under. Exhaling, push into Downward-Facing Dog Pose (*Adho Mukha Svanasana*).

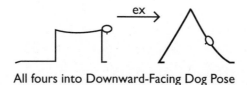

All fours into Downward-Facing Dog Pose

7d. Upward-Facing Dog Pose (*Urdhva Mukha Svanasana*)

From Downward-Facing Dog Pose (*Adho Mukha Svanasana*), inhale and swing into Upward-Facing Dog Pose (*Urdhva Mukha Svanasana*).

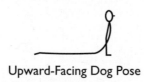

Upward-Facing Dog Pose

7e. Perform sequence in reverse

Go back through the sequence in reverse order. Exhale into Downward-Facing Dog Pose (*Adho Mukha Svanasana*). Inhale back onto all fours. Exhale into Child's Pose (*Balasana*). Inhale, coming back up to tall kneeling and lifting arms above the head; exhale and return the hands to the heart. Repeat the sequence 4 to 6 times. (If you prefer, it's fine to ignore the breathing guidance that's given for this sequence. Take extra breaths if you need to. Never strain with the breathing.)

8. Bow Pose variation (*Dhanurasana* variation)

Lie on your front with your arms by your sides. Inhaling, lift your chest as you bend both knees. Exhaling, lower the chest and straighten your legs back to the floor. Repeat 6 times, staying in the final pose for a few breaths.

Bow Pose variation

If you wish to work at a gentler level, skip step 9 and go straight to Sphinx Pose or repeat the Bow Pose variation once more.

9. Bow Pose (*Dhanurasana*)

Lie on your front, arms by your sides. Bend both knees and catch hold of your ankles. Lift your chest and knees up and away from the floor, gently pulling your shoulders back to open the chest. If comfortable, stay here for a few breaths. Then lower down to the floor, release the ankles, straighten your legs along the floor, and turn your head to one side, resting for a few breaths.

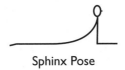

Bow Pose

10. Sphinx Pose (*Salamba Bhujangasana*)

Lying on your front, come up into a gentle backbend, propping yourself up on your fore-arms. Remember not to crease the back of the neck. Feel the tailbone and the crown of the head lengthening away from each other. Be aware of the natural rhythm of the breath. Stay here for a few breaths, silently repeating the affirmation: *My spacious heart holds all. My loving heart heals all.*

Sphinx Pose

11. Cat Pose (*Marjaryasana*) into Child's Pose (*Balasana*)

From all fours, exhale, lower the bottom to the heels and the head to the floor into Child's Pose (*Balasana*). Inhale and come back up to all fours. On each exhale chant aloud the mantra *Yam*. Repeat 8 times.

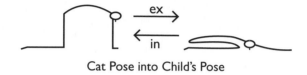

Cat Pose into Child's Pose

12. Child's Pose (*Balasana*)

Rest here for a few breaths here. If you are short of time, finish your practice here.

Child's Pose

13. Heart Chakra Meditation

If you have time, do the Heart Chakra Meditation that follows the overview of this practice. It can be done seated or lying down in Relaxation Pose (*Savasana*).

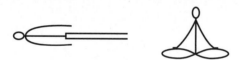

Heart Chakra Meditation

Heart Chakra Yoga Practice Overview

1. Heart Chakra Awareness Exercise

2. Knees-to-Chest Pose into leg raises × 6. Inhale: *My spacious heart holds all.* Exhale: *My loving heart heals all.*

3. Cat Pose into Child's Pose × 6

4. Mountain Pose. Inhale: *My spacious heart holds all.* Exhale: *My loving heart heals all.*

5. Warrior 1 variation and mantra *Yam* × 4. Repeat on other side.

6. Dancer Pose

7. Floor Salute to the Sun × 4–6

8. Bow Pose variation × 6. *For a gentler level, skip step 9 or repeat step 8.*

9. Bow Pose

10. Sphinx Pose. Affirm, *My spacious heart holds all. My loving heart heals all.*

11. Cat Pose into Child's Pose, with mantra *Yam* × 8

12. Child's Pose

13. Heart Chakra Meditation

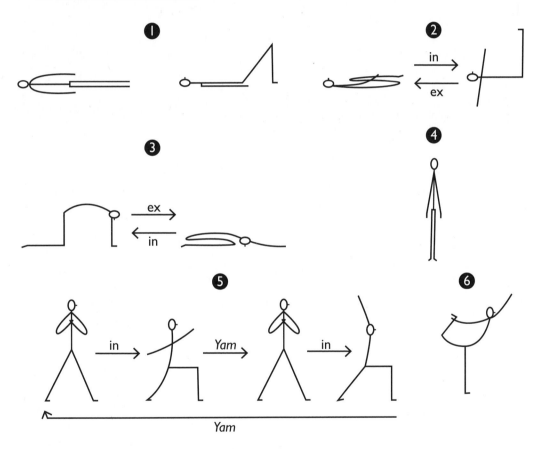

Heart Chakra Yoga Practice Overview

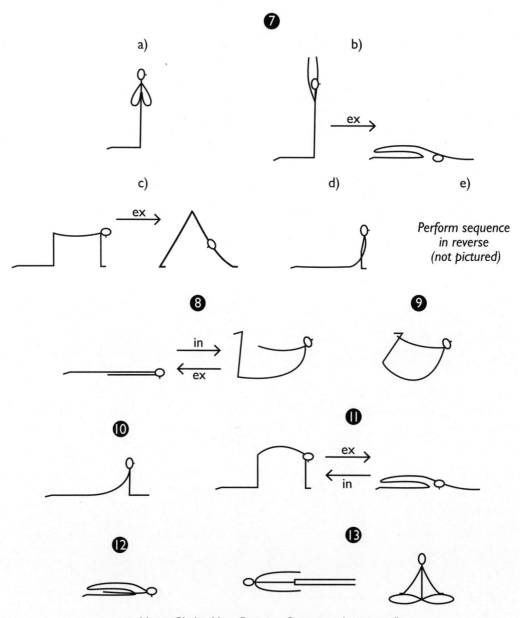

7

a)

b)

ex →

c)

ex →

d)

e)

*Perform sequence
in reverse
(not pictured)*

8

in →
← ex

9

10

11

ex →
← in

12

13

Heart Chakra Yoga Practice Overview (continued)

MEDITATION

Heart Chakra Meditation

This meditation can be used to begin or end a yoga practice, and it can also be used on its own as a standalone practice. The meditation engenders a sense of spaciousness and freedom. It's effective at shifting creative blocks, dispersing impatience, and engendering a receptive attitude that opens us to receiving inspiration.

The exercise can be done sitting or lying down. Allow 10 to 15 minutes.

Find yourself a comfortable position, either sitting or lying. If you are sitting, make sure you are sitting tall and symmetrically aligned around the center line of the body. If you are lying down, again make sure that you are symmetrically aligned.

Be aware of where the body is in contact with the earth beneath you and relax into that support. Be aware of the space around your body and feel yourself expanding into that space.

Bring your awareness to your heart center, silently repeat the heart chakra affirmation a few times:

Inhale: My spacious heart holds all.

Exhale: My loving heart heals all.

Then, let go of the affirmation and, keeping your awareness at the heart center, visualize a pink lotus flower on a bed of green leaves. Picture the color and shape of the flower. Notice whether it is open or in bud. Enjoy the serene beauty of the flower.

Now let go of picturing the flower and become aware of the natural flow of the breath, observing the breath without imposing a pattern on it. Notice the belly rising and falling and the chest expanding and condensing. Follow the full length of the in-breath and the full length of the out-breath. If your mind wanders off, just gently bring it back to riding the waves of the breath.

At the end of the next in-breath, observe there is a pause before you exhale, and at the end of the exhale, notice there is a pause before you inhale. Simply observe the pause and relax into it. There's no need to force it. Let it be easy and effortless. At the end of each exhale, consciously relax your belly, and allow the inhale to arise out of the pause, with no effort on your part. Create space and be inspired by the breath.

Now, keeping your awareness at the heart center, carry on observing the pauses between the breaths, and during the pause, silently say the mantra *Yam* (pronounced *yum*). Inhale, pause (*Yam*), exhale, pause (*Yam*). Repeat this over several breaths.

When you are ready, let go of repeating the mantra. Notice how you are feeling now. Resolve to take this loving, spacious feeling into the next thing that you do today.

MEDITATION

Heart Chakra Compassionate Walking Meditation

Whenever you have to walk anywhere, you can connect with your heart chakra simply by sending love and compassion to yourself and others as you walk. You can do this informally by simply smiling at passersby and silently sending them good wishes: "I hope you have a good day today." Or if you prefer, you can use formal loving kindness (*metta*) phrases as you walk:

May I be safe.
May I be happy.
May I be healthy.
May I live with ease.

You can strengthen your sense of connection with those you encounter by silently repeating phrases for both of you:

May you and I be happy.
May you and I live with ease.

You can also widen your circle of compassion by sending good wishes to animals, birds, trees, rocks, the sky, and the earth. To conclude your walking meditation, bring your awareness back to observing the sensations of your feet in contact with the earth as you walk. Thank the earth for supporting you during this walking meditation.

Heart Chakra Writing Meditation

For full instructions on how to do a writing meditation, go to the Writing Meditation with Focus section (see page 44).

Set your timer for 10 to 20 minutes and write meditatively on one or more of the following subjects:

- The infinite space of the heart.
- Freedom is…
- When heaven and earth are reunited…
- To mend a broken heart, you…
- Unconditional love means…

If writing isn't your thing, feel free to work with the above topics in any other medium. For example, paint a picture, make a collage, compose a song, or take some photos, working with the above themes.

Heart Chakra Meditation Questions

For full instructions on how to use the meditation questions, see page 47.

- How can I create balance between material and spiritual concerns in my life?
- What's the best way to cultivate compassion and kindness for myself and others?
- What emotions need to be brought to my heart for healing?
- How can I help to create a world that is just and fair for all?
- Am I creating space in my life for love to blossom?

CHAPTER 9

Communication Chakra
(Vishuddha)

Find Your Creative Voice

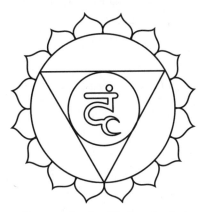

Communication Chakra Symbol

This chakra enables you to give voice to your creations and to communicate your vision. It teaches you to speak up and be heard but also to listen and learn. Working with this chakra teaches you to speak from the heart, to impart your wisdom through your creativity, and to receive wisdom through creative listening.

The Communication Chakra at a Glance

Sanskrit Name: *Vishuddha* (pure wheel)

Physical Location: Neck, throat, mouth, tongue, and ears

Element: Ether

Color: Blue

Yantra: A circle

Seed Mantra: *Ham* (pronounced *hum*)

Affirmations: *I speak my truth with love. I speak my truth with compassion.*

Main Creative Concerns: Giving voice to your creations, communicating your vision, speaking from the heart, imparting your wisdom through your creativity, and receiving wisdom through creative listening.

Balanced: Eloquent, authentic speaker, knows when to speak and when to remain silent, able to express emotions intelligently, good listener, capable of speaking truth to power, assertive, directs anger creatively, forthright.

Excessive: Verbose, dominates the conversation, a poor listener, uncomfortable with silence, overshares, emotions out of control, bullying tone, egocentric.

Deficient: Quiet, timid, unconfident speaker, represses emotions, unassertive, indirect, manipulates behind the scenes, bashful, a doormat, blocked creativity.

Life Issues: Communication, self-expression, emotional intelligence, assertiveness, truth telling, listening and learning, creativity.

Healing Practices: Self-expression, singing, chanting, pranayama, yoga, writing, any expressive and creative activities, public speaking, listening skills, talking therapies, any therapies that involve emotional release, truth telling, laughter, neck and shoulder massage, facial exercises, neck and shoulder exercises, assertiveness training.

Find Your Creative Voice

The communication chakra, at the throat, enables us to express ourselves clearly and authentically. It takes courage to give voice to our truth through our creative pursuits. However, the work we have done on the first four chakras will support us in this endeavor. When we listen to the wisdom of the heart chakra, we know when to speak and when to stay silent. The root chakra provides the stability and support we need to be able to risk speaking out. The sacral chakra at the belly puts us in touch with our gut feelings and helps us be clear about what we wish to express. The solar plexus chakra gives us the confidence to assert ourselves and to speak out.

If you are seeking to find your creative voice, then a good question to ask yourself is "What do I want to express?" Once you know what you want to give voice to, you will be more motivated to find a vehicle to express your vision. For example, I am driven to write by a sense of injustice. Ever since I was a child, I looked around and sensed that the world was not fair, and I wanted it to be fairer. As a child, I lived in fear because of the coercive control my father exerted over my mum and the rest of the family. This was very scary at times; however, I was never broken by the situation because I retained a sense of injustice and rebellion. This meant that although my life was never easy, my spirit stayed whole and intact. When I was a teenager, I discovered feminism, and with this came the realization that the reason my father was able to control the family in this way was due to a patriarchal system that reinforced this behavior in men and encouraged a submissive attitude in women. Consequently, feminism is a strong driving force underlying my desire to create and express myself.

Initially, my urge to write yoga books was driven by a desire to expose the sexism that seemed to be rife in the yoga world. I began a quest of finding out everything I could about the patriarchal roots of yoga. However, eventually an awareness arose in me that just cataloguing the chauvinism in yoga was a negative approach, and I wanted to counterpose that by also offering an alternative vison. I wanted to be part of creating a yoga that has the potential to be the balm that heals and makes us whole again regardless of our gender.

Speaking our truth, of course, can be a risky business. However, there are also risks incurred to our emotional and physical well-being from pushing down our truth and remaining silent. When we are in the habit of perpetually biting our tongue and suppressing our feelings, the cost will be a sense of constriction in the throat and the communication chakra. When there is a blockage in this chakra, all the other chakras are affected, and our vital energy is unable to flow freely. Everything flows better, including our creativity, when we create an outlet for our feelings by expressing them in words that are authentic and ring true.

Words are powerful. Words have the power to create and to destroy. When you work with this chakra, it pays to take some time to consider what is it that you wish to express. Connect to your heart. What matters to you? What moves you? What bugs you so much that it motivates you to power up your creativity to create change? Be authentic. Don't just jump on a popular bandwagon; channel your energy into expressing your own unique vision. If you do this, others will naturally listen to and respond to what you have to say.

Speak with Love, Listen with Compassion

There is an active and receptive ebb and flow to creativity. We give of ourselves to the world through our self-expression. This is the active phase of creativity. And then we nourish our creativity by listening to our own inner wisdom and to what others have to say. This is the receptive phase of creativity. The self-expression associated with the communication chakra must be balanced by its more subtle partner, which is the ability to listen and learn. Sometimes it is good to express yourself and make your voice heard, at other times it's better to stay silent and listen. It can be empowering to share your own experience, but it's also important to listen to what others have to say. Self-expression will be wiser and kinder if it is moderated by listening to the wisdom of the heart. When our self-expression is heart-centered, we are in a better position to intuit when to speak and when to remain silent.

We live in a noisy age of social media in which we are rewarded for always having an opinion, and the noisiest, most outraged opinions get the most oxygen. Sometimes it's good to turn off your phone, to disconnect from the echo chamber of social media, and to reconnect with the tangible, natural world around you. The internet can be an asset and a great way of sharing your creativity and connecting with others. However, we can fritter away our creative expression on chasing online "likes" with posts that are ephemeral and short lived.

Words can bring us closer together, and words can divide us. Can you put your own opinions aside and listen to what someone else has to say? Are you frightened of silence? Do you always have to fill in the gaps of a conversation? Can you learn to relax into and be comfortable with silence? You can use that quiet space to listen to yourself and others. Sacred sound emerges out of the silence. Sometimes fear leads us to remain silent. At other times it is wisdom that prompts us not to speak. The value of silence is that if we say less, often others will say more. When was the last time someone gave you a good listening to? Feeling heard by others validates our experience and is therapeutic. Conversely, we feel devalued and disheartened when we sense we are not being listened to.

Creative listening is an art. It involves active listening, noticing the speaker's tone of voice, hearing what is said behind the words, and picking up on the emotions beneath the words. You encourage the speaker to open up and to share more by asking open questions, and if you repeat back to the person what you think you have heard them say, they will feel listened to and heard. As you listen, stay aware of the thoughts and feelings that their words evoke in you. Resist the urge to jump in immediately with a retort. Notice when you stop listening to what they are saying and start preparing your response.

Our yoga practice teaches us to rehearse the process of deep listening, which in turn benefits our creativity. We always commence our yoga practice by listening. We tune in to our body, we observe our thoughts, we become aware of our emotional state, we listen to our breath. Throughout our practice we continually return to this act of listening and responding to the body, the mind, and breath. It is this receptive state induced by yoga that creates the space within for us to be able to hear the small, still voice of inspiration when it calls. We allow inner prompts to guide us which poses we should do and when to push harder or to work more gently. All these listening skills that we cultivate in our yoga practice prepare us for the same deep listening that we need to call upon when we are involved in creative activities.

I attended a Quaker meeting for a number of years, and although I am not a Quaker, it has influenced the way that I approach my writing and my yoga. Quaker meetings begin with those assembled sitting in silence, silently listening for the voice of the spirit, and only speaking when the spirit moves them to do so. When I write, I always begin with a period of silent listening. I wait for the spirit to move me before I write. I do the same with my home yoga practice. I wait and listen for the prompts of the spirit to guide me concerning which yoga poses to do. I do the same when I am teaching a yoga class: I watch the class; listen to how they are responding; listen to my own emotions, thoughts, and physical sensations; and shape the class practice accordingly. For me "spirit" is not attached to any religion. It is my individual spirit, it is also the collective spirit of humanity, and it is possibly a universal spirit that pervades all things both animate and inanimate. However, you can adapt this approach to fit in with your own belief system, and you can tap into an infinite source of inspiration by learning to listen well.

Yoga Inspired by the Communication Chakra

When working with the communication chakra, we center our awareness in the neck, throat, the mouth, and the ears. At times when we are emotionally blocked, the throat can feel constricted. So we use the color blue and the element ether, which are both associated with the chakra, to create a blue-sky spacious awareness in the practice, to release constriction and engender a sense of freedom.

This is the chakra to work with if you are having difficulty expressing yourself. You can overcome this block by the use of sound and mantra in your practice, which gets you in the habit of making yourself heard! We can use sound in a way that is freeing and exhilarating, as well as safe and enjoyable for releasing pent-up energy and ridding yourself of frustration. We can also integrate simple mantras into flowing yoga sequences (*vinyasas*).

We create equilibrium in the communication chakra by balancing self-expression with listening. We listen to and meditate upon the sounds around us and the sound of the breath. We cultivate an awareness of the silence that all sounds arise from and return to.

Communication Chakra Yoga Practice

This is the go-to practice when you feel creatively blocked and want to get your ideas flowing again. The practice is cleansing, calming, uplifting, and engenders a sense of emotional release. We use sound in the practice to encourage self-expression, and, in contrast, we use silence to encourage a receptive state of mind, open to receiving fresh inspiration.

The affirmation we use in the practice is *I speak my truth with love*. We coordinate it with the breath in this way:

Inhale: Loving heart

Exhale: Truthful speech

Allow 20 to 30 minutes.

At the end of these instructions, you'll find an illustrated aide-mémoire for the whole practice.

1. Communication Chakra Awareness Exercise

Find yourself a comfortable sitting position. Bring your awareness to your neck, the throat, the mouth, the back of the throat, and the ears.

Notice any sounds that you can hear inside and outside the room. Be aware of the soundscape around you.

Now bring your awareness to the natural flow of your breath. Be aware of the sound of the breath. Then, each time you breathe out, make a humming sound. Repeat for several breaths. Then, stop humming and be aware of the effect that the vibration of the humming has had upon you.

Communication Chakra Awareness Exercise

2. Cat Pose (*Marjaryasana*) into Child's Pose (*Balasana*)

From all fours, hum the breath out as you lower the bottom to the heels and the head to the floor into Child's Pose (*Balasana*). Inhale and come back up to all fours. Repeat 8 times.

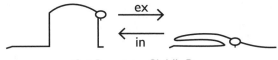

Cat Pose into Child's Pose

3. *Ha* breath

Stand in Mountain Pose (*Tadasana*). Inhale, taking both arms out to the side at just below shoulder height. Exhale, making a *Ha* sound as you bend the knees, lean slightly forward, and bring both hands to the belly. Return to the starting position on the inhale. Repeat 3 to 6 times.

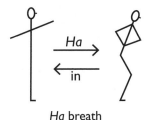

Ha breath

4. Lion Pose (*Simhasana*)

Take the legs 2 to 3 feet apart, toes turned slightly out. Bend your arms and make tight fists with your hands. Screw up your face, eyes shut tight. Exhale, bend the knees, lean slightly forward, and open your mouth wide as you stretch out your tongue, making a *ha* sound as you expel the breath. At the same time, open your eyes wide and spread your fingers wide. Inhaling, straighten the legs and come back to the starting position with clenched fists. Repeat 4 times.

Lion Pose

5. Warrior 1 (*Virabhadrasana* 1) variation

Stand tall with your feet hip width apart, turn your left foot slightly out, and take a big step forward with your right leg. Place your hands on your belly. Inhaling, bend your right knee, opening your arms out wide to the side. Exhaling, straighten your right leg and bring your hands back to your belly. Coordinate the breath with the mantra *Ma*. Inhale, and on each exhale chant *Ma*. Do 6 repetitions on this side and then repeat on the other side.

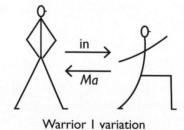

Warrior 1 variation

6. Wood-Chop Squat with *Ha* breathing

Stand with your feet parallel, shoulder width apart. Raise both arms above your head, fingertips touching. Bend your knees into a squat, keep your arms straight, and chop down, making a *Ha* sound on the out-breath. Inhale and come back to the starting position. Repeat 6 times.

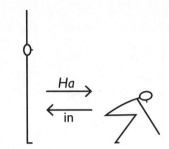

Wood-Chop Squat with *Ha* breathing

7. Child's Pose (*Balasana*) into Upward-Facing Dog Pose (*Urdhva Mukha Svanasana*)

From sitting kneeling, sit back into Child's Pose (*Balasana*), arms outstretched along the floor. Inhale, moving forward into Upward-Facing Dog (*Urdhva Mukha Svanasana*), arching your back and keeping your knees on the floor. Exhale back into Child's Pose. You can silently coordinate the breath with the affirmation. Inhale and affirm, *Loving heart*. Exhale and affirm, *Truthful speech*. Repeat 6 times as you move between the two poses.

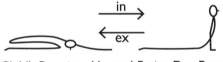

Child's Pose into Upward-Facing Dog Pose

8. Child's Pose (*Balasana*)

Rest for a few breaths here. Be particularly aware of the exhale, noticing the pause between each exhale and the next inhale. With each exhale feel yourself relaxing a little more deeply.

Child's Pose

9. Seated Forward Bend (*Paschimottanasana*) and mantra *Ram*

Sit tall, legs outstretched (bend the knees to ease the pose). Bring your awareness to the solar plexus. Inhale and raise the arms. Keeping your awareness at the solar plexus, exhale, and chant the mantra *Ram* (pronounced *rum*). At the end of the exhale, as you complete the chant, fold forward over the legs. Inhale and return to starting position. Repeat 6 times and on the final time stay for a few breaths in the Seated Forward Bend. Note: never strain with the breathing. Take extra breaths if you need to.

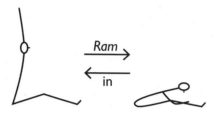

Seated Forward Bend and mantra *Ram*

10. *Ma-Om* kneeling sequence

Come to tall kneeling, hands in Prayer Position (*Namaste*). Inhale and raise arms. Exhaling, chant the mantra *Ma* as you fold forward into Child's Pose (*Balasana*), arms outstretched along the floor. Inhale and come onto all fours. On the exhale, chant *Om*, sit back into Child's Pose. Inhale and come back to tall kneeling with arms raised. Exhale and bring the hands into Prayer Position. Repeat the sequence 4 to 6 times.

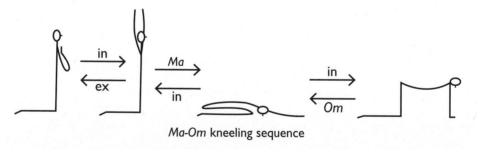

Ma-Om kneeling sequence

11. Mantra *Ma* and arm movements

Find a comfortable seated position. Rest your hands on your belly. Inhale and take your arms out to the side. Exhale and bring your hands back to the belly, chanting the mantra *Ma*. Stay for one breath, with the hands resting on the belly. Repeat 6 times.

If you are pushed for time, you can finish your practice here.

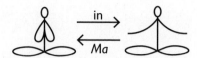

Mantra *Ma* and arm movements

12. Communication Chakra Meditation

If you have more time, spend a few minutes resting in the Relaxation Pose (*Savasana*), and then do the Communication Chakra Meditation, which follows the overview of this practice.

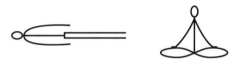

Savasana and Communication Chakra Meditation

Communication Chakra Yoga Practice Overview

1. Communication Chakra Awareness Exercise

2. Cat Pose into Child's Pose with humming × 8

3. *Ha* breath × 3–6

4. Lion Pose × 4

5. Warrior 1 variation with mantra *Ma* × 6. Repeat on other side.

6. Wood-Chop Squat with *Ha* breathing × 6

7. Child's Pose into Upward-Facing Dog × 6. Inhale: *Loving heart*. Exhale: *Truthful speech*.

8. Child's Pose. Rest.

9. Seated Forward Bend with mantra *Ram* × 6

10. *Ma-Om* kneeling sequence, × 4–6

11. Mantra *Ma* and arm movements × 6. *End here if short of time.*

12. Communication Chakra Meditation

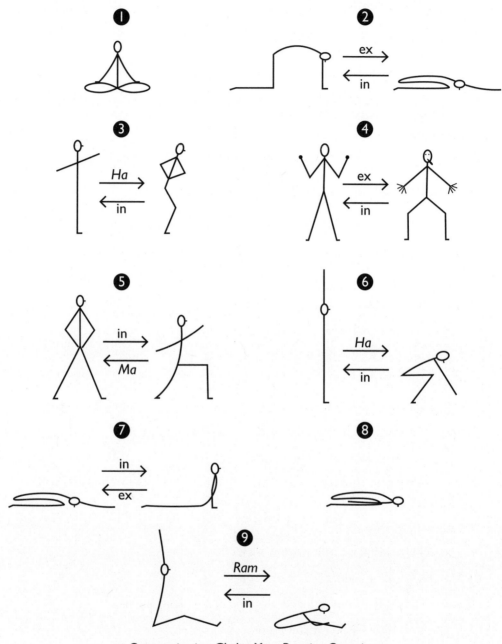

Communication Chakra Yoga Practice Overview

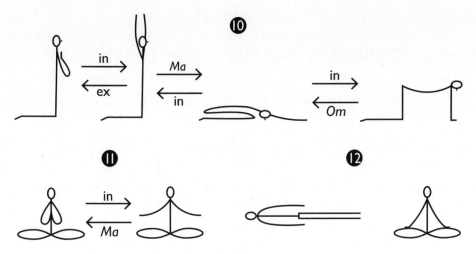

Communication Chakra Yoga Practice Overview (continued)

MEDITATION

Communication Chakra Meditation

This meditation can be used to begin or end a yoga practice, and it can also be used on its own as a standalone practice. The meditation is calming and uplifting, and it engenders a sense of freedom and spaciousness. It teaches us to balance self-expression with listening.

Allow 10 to 15 minutes.

Find yourself a comfortable sitting position. Bring your awareness to the neck, throat, mouth, back of the throat, and ears. Notice any sounds that you can hear inside the room and outside the room. Sounds near and sounds far away. Notice the silent spaces between the sounds. Notice how sounds arise and pass away.

Now bring your awareness to the natural flow of your breath. Be aware of the sound of the breath. Then on each exhale, make a humming sound. Repeat for several breaths. When you have stopped humming, be aware of the effect the vibration of the humming has had upon you. Notice the silence and the sounds that arise out of and return to the silence.

Then, once again bring your awareness to the throat and visualize the color blue, which is the color associated with this chakra. Aim to cultivate a sense of freedom and spaciousness by visualizing the blue of the ocean, a clear blue sky, a field of blue cornflowers, or any other image that appeals to you.

Now let go of this image but retain that sense of openness. Silently repeat the communication chakra affirmation a few times: *I speak my truth with love.*

When you are ready, let go of repeating the affirmation. Notice how you are feeling. Resolve to balance loving speech and respectful listening in all your encounters today.

MEDITATION

Communication Chakra Mindfulness of Sound Walking Meditation

This meditation can be done inside or outside. It takes about 5 to 10 minutes. It is a wonderful way of connecting with the environment around you and increasing your power of observation. If, like me, you live in the city, you might find that you have developed a habit of cutting off and zoning out intrusive urban sounds, in which case you will need to reverse this habit and lean into the sounds around you during this meditation. It's always good to challenge our *samskaras* (habits), and for a creative person it's important to be in touch with all your senses.

To do this meditation, simply be aware of the soundscape around you as you walk. Listen to the sound of your feet as they strike the ground. Notice how the sound of your footsteps varies depending on what surface you are on: a soft sound on grass, a heavy sound on concrete, and so on. Be aware of natural sounds: leaves crackling underfoot, birdsong, children playing, the whistle of the wind through the trees, water flowing. Be aware of manmade sounds: a train pulling out of the station, a bike whizzing by, the purr of a car's engine, the dull throb of heavy traffic. Notice how sounds arise and pass away. Be aware of any tendency you have to judge sounds. Cultivate a non-judgmental attitude, neither seeking sounds out nor pushing them away.

To conclude your walking meditation, let go of observing sounds and return to a more general awareness of your surroundings. Be aware of your feet and the contact they make with the earth with each step. Notice how the meditation has affected you and any changes it has brought about in how you are feeling physically, mentally, and emotionally today.

MEDITATION

Communication Chakra Writing Meditation

For full instructions on how to do a writing meditation, go to the Writing Meditation with Focus section (see page 44).

Set your timer for 10 to 20 minutes and write meditatively on one or more of the following subjects:

- What I want to say is…

- Blue

- Write a letter to a person in your life whom you find difficult. Write freely; do not censor yourself. Once you have completed your writing, read it through, then tear it up, burn it, compost it, or dispose of it in another way! Seriously, don't send it!

- Imagine yourself in the shoes of the person you find difficult. Now, write a letter, in the first person, as if you are that person writing to you.

- Silence is…

Communication Chakra Meditation Questions

For full instructions on how to use the meditation questions, see page 47.

- What is my predominant emotion today, and what is the best way to express it?

- What skills would I need to acquire to become a good listener?

- Whom do I admire as an orator, and what is it about their speech that pleases me?

- What do I wish to express through my creativity (art, poetry, writing, painting, etc.)?

- What three truths would I most like to tell? And whom would I tell them to?

CHAPTER 10

Third Eye Chakra
(Ajna)

Sharpen Your Inner Vision

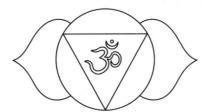

Third Eye Chakra Symbol

Working with this chakra develops your intuition, clairvoyance, and imagination. You learn to see with your inner eye, to visualize what it is you wish to create, and to remember your dreams and be guided by them. Your creative vision is illuminated, and you are open to receiving inspiration from above. You see and you know.

The Third Eye Chakra at a Glance

Sanskrit Name: *Ajna* (command wheel)

Physical Location: Above and between the eyebrows

Element: Light

Color: Indigo

Yantra: A crescent moon above a downward-pointing triangle, containing the *Om* symbol, all enclosed within a two-petaled circle

Seed Mantra: *Am* or *Om*

Affirmations: *Love flows. Light heals. Love lights my way.*

Main Creative Concerns: Learning to see with the inner eye and visualizing what you wish to create. Developing imagination, accessing the dreamworld of the subconscious, and opening yourself to receive inspiration. Bringing your creations out into the light. Making creative leaps of faith, guided by your intuition.

Balanced: Intuitive, clear-sighted, a beacon of light to others, imaginative, visionary, spiritual but grounded, perceptive, remembers dreams, sees the bigger picture and takes care of the details, clear judgment, sees beyond superficial appearances, appreciates beauty.

Excessive: Cerebral, floaty, spiritual zealot, evangelical, nervy, poor psychic boundaries, superstitious, abstract thinker, ungrounded, flowery, impractical.

Deficient: Superficial, unperceptive, unimaginative, unspiritual, ultra-practical, cynical, materialistic, lack of foresight, poor intuition.

Life Issues: Balancing the spiritual and material aspects of life, learning to trust your own judgment, developing emotional intelligence. If there is a history of abuse, ensuring that the third eye is not overdeveloped at the expense of the chakras below. Ensuring that you have developed the stability and support of the lower chakras in order to be able to work on this chakra safely.

Healing Practices: Relaxation, meditation, yoga nidra, eye exercises, finding the support of a well-grounded spiritual community, keeping a dream diary, prayer, yoga, guided visualizations, reading fiction (which encourages visualizing fictional scenes in your head), moonlit walks, stargazing, intuitive astrology, astronomy, all imaginative creative pursuits.

Dream Your Creations into Being

Light is the "element" associated with this chakra, and so for those involved in creative pursuits, working with the chakra can be illuminating and rewarding. This chakra has an aura of mystery about it because it enables us to see with the inner eye and to peep behind the veil of everyday reality. However, on a more mundane level, we shouldn't overlook the benefits of mindfully looking with our two actual eyes and fully appreciating the beauty of the world around us, which often goes unnoticed when we are on autopilot.

The ability to see with the inner eye and to perceive the essence that lies behind material reality is an indispensable skill for the creative person. Paul Gauguin, the painter, said, "I shut my eyes in order to see."[30] With the inner eye we can picture what we would like to make manifest, and it is this that makes the third eye chakra such a potent ally on our creative journey.

Artists often express something that is just out of sight for the rest of us, and their work is a revelation helping others see more clearly. The beat generation writer Jack Kerouac wrote, "The jewel center of interest is the eye within the eye."[31] And so it is that the third eye chakra enables us to look beyond appearances and to see what lies beneath the surface. When this chakra is activated, it opens us to a deep source of intuitive wisdom, which can help us to make wise and insightful choices during the creative process. Regardless of whether you are involved in the arts or the sciences, working with this chakra opens you to the possibility of making creative leaps of intuition, resulting in innovation.

In yogic states of deep relaxation, you are more open to receive the surreal, creative pairings and paradoxes that the subconscious mind delights in and that give an edge to creativity. Your relaxed mind is a deep pool, and you are a diver who can plumb the depths of the subconscious mind and access the symbols, dreams, and archetypes that reside there. One of the gifts of my daily early morning yoga practice is that fragments of forgotten dreams often float to the surface of my mind. Later I jot them down in a dream diary, and that helps me identify themes and symbols that recur in my dreams. Our dreams can reveal the path that leads to the pot of gold at the end of the rainbow.

---

30. Paul Gauguin, "Paul Gauguin's Quotes," Gauguin.org, 2021, https://www.gauguin.org/quotes.jsp.
31. Jack Kerouac, "Belief and Technique for Modern Prose," *Evergreen Review* 2, no. 8 (spring 1959): 57.

In sutra 3:33 Patanjali states, "From intuition, one knows everything."[32] The ancient Tantric yogis combined scientific self-observation with an astonishingly creative approach that enabled them to intuit, through the power of imagination and visualization, the network of the subtle energy system and how it manifested within the body. The Tantric yogi turned his gaze inward, exploring his body and mapping out the anatomy of the astral or subtle body. This is relevant to those involved in creative pursuits because the ancient yogis show us that it is possible, through a creative leap of intuition and imagination, to construct the entire universe within our own body. By mastering the art of visualizing the creative power within your body, you are rehearsing the power of embodying that force of creativity in the wider world.

Extraordinary Powers to Be Handled with Care

The yoga sage Patanjali, in his Yoga Sutra, describes the extraordinary powers (*siddhis*), that the yogi can acquire through a dedicated practice. These include invisibility, super-human strength, knowledge of past and future lives, and exceptional states of consciousness. He also warns about the dangers of getting seduced by these extraordinary powers and considers them as a worldly distraction on the path, rather than a final destination.[33]

If you have been practicing yoga for a while, you might have noticed how yoga has sharpened your intuition, even to the point of clairvoyance. However, a difficulty can arise as sometimes people who are emotionally unbalanced are attracted to the drama of developing the clairvoyant powers of the third eye chakra, and this can be detrimental if the lower chakras are unable to support this surge in psychic power. Another consideration is that for some people the third eye chakra might be overdeveloped, whereas the lower chakras are underdeveloped. This is especially noticeable in those who have experienced childhood trauma.

In meditation, our mind is calm like a pool, and within that pool we see ourselves and our lives reflected back to us as they really are, and this can be both beautiful and disturbing. Working with the third eye chakra is warrior work, and it is vitally important that you have done the groundwork of working with the lower chakras first, to give you the support, stability, and the resilience that you need to work responsibly with this chakra. The great thing about exploring the chakras through a physical yoga practice is that it

---

32. Barbara Stoler Miller, trans., *Yoga: Discipline of Freedom; The Yoga Sutra Attributed to Patanjali* (New York: Bantam Books, 1998), 67.

33. Stoler Miller, trans., *Yoga: Discipline of Freedom*, 68.

keeps you grounded in your body, and this is particularly relevant when working with the third eye chakra.

When we enter a state of deep, yogic relaxation, we open to the possibility of being gifted a healing symbol to work with. It is the inner eye that reveals the symbol to us, which is oftentimes the medicine that we need to heal. Several years ago, this happened to me when I was going through a particularly difficult time. A much-loved member of my family was struggling with their mental health, and frustratingly, everything I tried to help seemed to make matters worse. One day, I sat down to meditate and somehow, despite the constant worry of that time, I managed to drop into a very relaxed state. In this meditative state, an image floated into my mind of what I later realized was a painting by Holman Hunt called *The Light of the World*. The painting depicts Jesus, a halo of light around his head, holding a lantern in his hand and knocking at a door, deep within a forest. Interestingly, although I don't consider myself a Christian, I found this peaceful image helped me feel supported in my troubles and surrounded by love. Fortunately, over time I managed to connect with my loved one, and they eventually made a full recovery.

Another consideration for the creative person is that when we are immersed in a project, we spend a lot of time visualizing with the inner eye what it is we wish to create, and this can result in our living in a dream world, with our energy over-focused in our head. It's a good idea to counterpose this with the grounding, centering activities associated with the lower chakras, such as being outside in daylight (rather than tethered to the computer), gardening, baking, and connecting with friends. It's tempting to skip these activities, especially when you are working to a creative deadline; however, it pays dividends to intersperse the intensity of the creative process with these more worldly activities. You will feel better, and it keeps you and your work fresher. Right … paragraph finished … so, please excuse me while I pop outside into the garden to sweep up some autumn leaves on the path.

Yoga Inspired by the Third Eye Chakra

As already stated, when working with the third eye chakra, it's important to stay grounded and centered, and you can do this by integrating your work on this chakra into a physical yoga practice. In a third eye yoga practice, we aim to balance a focus on the third eye by simultaneously focusing on the sacral chakra at the belly. Both are centers of deep inner wisdom, intuition, seeing, and knowing. The sacral chakra is one step away from the root chakra and earth; the third eye chakra is one step away from the crown chakra and heaven. The sacral chakra is concerned with wisdom on an earthly plain, and the third eye chakra with heavenly wisdom.

The "element" associated with the third eye chakra is light, and it can be pleasurable and illuminating to introduce imagery of light into your yoga practice.

Through the use of mantra, we can experience vibration at the third eye, particularly during the prolonged *mm* sound of the mantra *Ma* and the mantra *Om*. Interestingly, the mother syllable *Maa* in ancient Egyptian hieroglyphics meant "to see."[34] *Ma* is a wonderfully nurturing mantra to introduce into a third eye chakra yoga practice and is also another good way of grounding yourself when working with this chakra.

To activate the inner eye, it's helpful to visualize colors, light, yantras, and mandalas, as part of a meditation or visualization.

Third Eye Chakra Yoga Practice

This practice is energizing, lightens your mood, unblocks stuck energy, and induces a sense of clarity. By balancing our focus on the third eye chakra, with a complimentary focus on the sacral chakra at the belly, we stay grounded and avoid getting spaced-out.

The affirmation we use in the practice is *Love flows. Light heals.* We coordinate it with the breath in this way:

Inhale: Love flows.

Exhale: Light heals.

Allow 20 to 30 minutes.

At the end of these instructions, you'll find an illustrated aide-mémoire for the whole practice.

---

34. Walker, *The Woman's Encyclopedia of Myths and Secrets*, 294.

1. Third Eye Chakra Awareness Exercise

Find a comfortable seated position. Bring your awareness to the third eye chakra, between the brows, and as you hold your awareness here, become aware of the natural flow of your breath. Then silently repeat the third eye chakra affirmation a few times. Inhale and affirm, *Love flows.* Exhale and affirm, *Light heals.*

Third Eye Chakra Awareness Exercise

2. Mantra *Ma* and arm movements

In a seated position, rest your hands on your belly. Inhale and take your arms out to the side. Exhale and bring your hands back to the belly, chanting the mantra *Ma* (*mm-ah*). Repeat 6 times.

Please note: we divide the mantra *Ma* into two syllables, *mm* and *ah*. Making a prolonged *mm* sound, direct your awareness to the third eye chakra, between the brows, and making a prolonged *ah* sound, direct awareness to the sacral chakra at the belly.

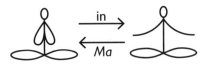

Mantra *Ma* and arm movements

3. Dynamic Horse Pose (*Vatayanasana*) variation

Stand with the legs apart, toes turned slightly out. Take both arms out to the side and above your head, bringing the hands together. Exhaling, bend both knees as if you were sitting down on a high stool, and bring the hands to the heart in prayer position. Inhaling, straighten the legs, taking arms out to the side and above the head, back to the starting position. You can silently coordinate the breath with the affirmation. On each inhale affirm, *Love flows.* On each exhale affirm, *Light heals.* Repeat 8 times. On the final time stay for a few breaths in the Dynamic Horse Pose (*Vatayanasana*) variation, bringing your awareness to the third eye chakra.

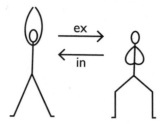

Dynamic Horse Pose variation

4. Eagle Pose (*Garudasana*)

Stand in Mountain Pose (*Tadasana*). Bend your knees, raise your left foot up, cross your left thigh over your right, and, if you can, hook the top of the left foot behind the lower right calf (for an easier option, stay in Mountain Pose and just do the arm movements). Extend both arms out in front, parallel to the floor. Place the right arm over the left, bend the elbows, nestling the right elbow into the crook of the left, and bring the backs of the hands together or clasp the palms together. Gently raise the elbows a little, keeping the shoulders down and creating length in the back of the neck. Stay for a few breaths, directing your awareness to the third eye chakra. Repeat on the other side.

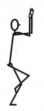

Eagle Pose

5. Opening and closing doors

Stand with the legs 2 to 3 feet apart, toes turned slightly out. Take the arms out to the sides at shoulder height and bend them, forming a right angle at the elbow, fingers pointing up toward the ceiling and palms facing forward. Exhale, bend the knees, and bring the forearms and hands together in front of the chest (doors closed). Inhale, straighten the legs, and "open the doors" by bringing the arms back to the starting position. Repeat 6 times.

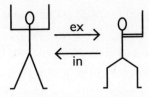

Opening and closing doors

6. Lunge Pose with arm movements (*Anjaneyasana* variation)

Come to tall kneeling. Take your right foot forward and bend the knee, bringing the knee over the ankle. Rest your fingertips lightly on your ears, elbows out to the side. Exhale, bringing the elbows to point to the front and down, rounding the upper back, and looking down. Inhaling, open the elbows, lift the chest, and look up slightly. Repeat 4 times and then stay in the open-chest position for a few breaths. Repeat on the other side.

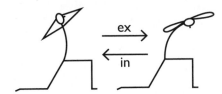

Lunge Pose with arm movements

7. Puppy Dog Pose (*Uttana Shishosana*) into Child's Pose (*Balasana*)

Come onto all fours. Walk the hands forward along the floor until your arms, head, and torso form one long diagonal line, keeping the thighs at a 90-degree angle. Keep the ears between the arms. Stay here for a few breaths. Then bend the knees, sit the bottom back onto the heels, and rest for a few breaths in Child's Pose (*Balasana*).

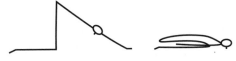

Puppy Dog Pose into Child's Pose

8. Child's Pose (*Balasana*) into Upward-Facing Dog Pose (*Urdhva Mukha Svanasana*)
From Child's Pose (*Balasana*) stretch the arms out along the floor. Inhale, moving forward into Upward-Facing Dog Pose (*Urdhva Mukha Svanasana*), arching your back, and keeping your knees on the floor. Exhale back into Child's Pose. You can silently coordinate the breath with the affirmation. Inhale and affirm, *Love flows*. Exhale and affirm, *Light heals*. Repeat 6 times as you move between the two poses.

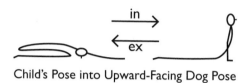

Child's Pose into Upward-Facing Dog Pose

9. Downward-Facing Dog Pose (*Adho Mukha Svanasana*)
From the all-fours position, turn the toes under and come into Downward-Facing Dog Pose (*Adho Mukha Svanasana*). Stay here for a few breaths and then lower down, coming to sitting, ready for the next pose. (More experienced students might wish to substitute a more advanced inverted pose here.)

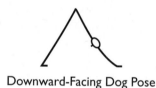

Downward-Facing Dog Pose

10. Seated Twist variation (*Ardha Matsyendrasana*)
Come to a seated position, legs outstretched. Bend your right knee and place your right foot on the outside of your left knee. Sit up tall, wrap your left arm around your right knee, and hug the knee into your chest. Place your right palm down on the floor behind you. Inhale, lengthen up through your spine, exhale, and twist, looking over your right shoulder. Stay in the twist, dropping your awareness down to your belly. Each time you exhale, gently pull in your lower abs and silently repeat the mantra *Vam*. Stay for a few breaths and then repeat on the other side. (More experienced students might wish to substitute a more complex seated twist here.)

Seated Twist variation

11. Seated Forward Bend (*Paschimottanasana*)

Sit tall, legs outstretched (bend the knees to ease the pose). Inhale and raise your arms. Exhale and fold forward over the legs. Inhale and return to starting position. You can silently coordinate the breath and movement with the affirmation. Inhale and affirm, *Love flows.* Exhale and affirm, *Light heals.* Repeat 6 times, and on the final time stay for a few breaths in the pose.

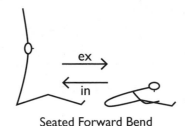

Seated Forward Bend

12. Mantra *Ma* and arm movements

We finish the practice as we began it with the mantra *Ma*. Come to a seated position and rest your hands on your belly. Inhale and take your arms out to the side. Exhale and bring your hands back to the belly, chanting the mantra *Ma* (*mm-ah*). Repeat 6 times. As before, we divide the mantra *Ma* into two syllables, *Mm* and *ah*. Making a prolonged *mm* sound, direct awareness to the third eye chakra, between the brows, and making a prolonged *ah* sound, direct awareness to the sacral chakra at the belly.

   If you wish, you can finish your practice here.

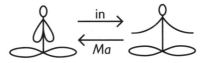

Mantra *Ma* and arm movements

13. Third Eye Chakra Circulating Light Visualization

If you have more time, then come into the Relaxation Pose (*Savasana*) for the Third Eye Chakra Circulating Light Visualization that follows the overview of this practice.

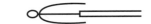

Third Eye Chakra Circulating Light Visualization

Third Eye Chakra Yoga Practice Overview

1. Third Eye Chakra Awareness Exercise

2. Mantra *Ma* and arm movements × 6

3. Dynamic Horse Pose × 8. Inhale: *Love flows.* Exhale: *Light heals.*

4. Eagle Pose

5. Opening and closing doors × 6

6. Lunge Pose with arm movements × 4 each side

7. Puppy Dog Pose into Child's Pose

8. Child's Pose into Upward-Facing Dog Pose × 6. Inhale: *Love flows.* Exhale: *Light heals.*

9. Downward-Facing Dog Pose

10. Seated Twist variation and mantra *Vam*

11. Seated Forward Bend × 6. Inhale: *Love flows.* Exhale: *Light heals.*

12. Mantra *Ma* with arm movements × 6. *If short of time, end here.*

13. Third Eye Chakra Circulating Light Visualization

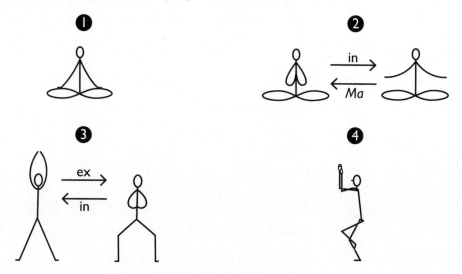

Third Eye Chakra Yoga Practice Overview

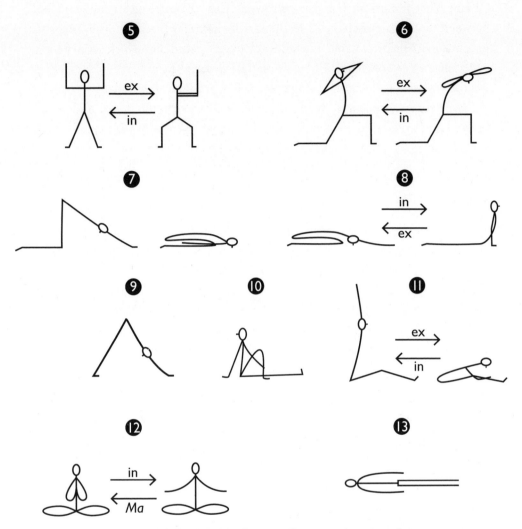

Third Eye Chakra Yoga Practice Overview (continued)

Third Eye Chakra Circulating Light Visualization

This meditation can be used to begin or end a yoga practice, and it can also be used on its own as a standalone practice. Light is the element associated with this chakra, and so we visualize light circulating around the body, which has an energizing effect, unblocking stuck, stagnant energy and encouraging a healthy, vibrant flow of prana, or chi. During the meditation, we create an energetic link between the third eye chakra and the sacral chakra at the belly. This keeps us grounded and helps us avoid any tendency to get spaced out, which some people experience when concentrating solely on the third eye chakra.

The exercise can be done sitting or lying down. Allow 10 minutes.

Bring your awareness to the third eye chakra, between the brows, and as you hold your awareness here, become aware of the natural flow of your breath. Then silently repeat the third eye chakra affirmation a few times:

Inhale: Love flows.

Exhale: Light heals.

Now, drop your awareness down to the lower belly, the sacral chakra, and imagine a ball of pure white light glowing here. Then visualize that you are circulating this ball of light down around the pelvic floor to the base of the spine, up through the center of the spine to the crown of the head, and then to the space between the brows, the third eye chakra. Pause briefly here and then take the light energy down the front of the spine and back to the lower belly again. Continue circulating the light in this loop of energy around the body.

If you are new to this visualization, you might prefer to let the breathing take care of itself. Once you have gained confidence, you can add a breathing pattern. On the inhale you direct the ball of light from the lower belly around and up the back of the body to between the brows, pausing briefly here, and then exhale, taking the light down the front of the body and back to the lower belly, pausing briefly here. Carry on breathing and visualizing the light circulating in a loop around the front and back of the body. Eventually, it will feel like it is the breath powering the light around the body.

When you feel ready, let go of circulating light around the body and allow your awareness first to rest at the space between the brows, and then drop it down to rest in the lower belly. Notice how the belly rises and falls with each in- and out-breath. Maintain your attention on the rising and falling of the belly and let go of everything else. Allow yourself to breathe and to simply be.

When you are ready, let go of following the breath. Become aware of bodily sensations, particularly noticing the sensations associated with where your body is in contact with the floor or your support. Observe what effect this visualization has had upon you. Do any movements you need to do to wake yourself up.

MEDITATION

Third Eye Chakra Appreciative, Slow Walking Meditation

In this meditation we slow our walking right down and take time to stop and appreciate the beauty all around us. If possible, do the meditation in a park or your garden, or go up a hill or into a forest. However, although natural surroundings are the ideal environment for this meditation, it can be done anywhere, even in an urban setting, as long as we pay attention and absorb all the details of the world around us through our eyes. The main purpose of the meditation is to encourage a meditative gaze, breaking the habit of thinking that we "know" an object and consequently not really seeing it in its full glory.

Allow 5 to 15 minutes.

We begin the meditation by slowing down our walking and being aware of the contact our feet are making with the earth with every step. Take time to look around you, taking in the details of your environment. If something catches your attention, stop to really look at it. Perhaps you notice the sun on a flower, and looking closely, you're amazed at the intricacy of the stamens inside. Or walking by water, you might stop to look, and on closer inspection, your eyes alight on tiny fishes darting about beneath the surface of the water. Even in the city, nature is always present, and you might spot a flower bursting through the tarmac, crimson autumn leaves blown in the wind along the pavement, or impressive cloud shapes racing across the sky. Even spending a few minutes gazing closely at a patch of grass will reveal a world within a world, a microcosm within the macrocosm.

If, like me, you are usually a brisk walker, initially it might be challenging for you to slow down. However, give it a try because this type of mindful walking is beneficial for your health, lowering your blood pressure and slowing down your heart rate, and it improves your mental health and sense of well-being.[35] You could always make a compromise and do five minutes of this slow, appreciative walking at the beginning and end of a brisker walk. Also, your creativity benefits

---

35. Michael Mosley, "Green Spaces," *Just One Thing*, BBC Radio, May 9, 2021, radio broadcast, 15:00, https://www.bbc.co.uk/programmes/m000vy1l.

from this honing of your observation skills, opening yourself up to a beautiful world that you wouldn't get to see on autopilot.

MEDITATION

Third Eye Chakra Writing Meditation

For full instructions on how to do a writing meditation, go to the Writing Meditation with Focus section (see page 44).

Set your timer for 10 to 20 minutes and write meditatively on one of the following subjects:

- The inner eye sees...
- The landscape of dreams
- To me, beauty is...
- Intuition
- My peaceful place

Third Eye Chakra Meditation Questions

For full instructions on how to use the meditation questions, see page 47.

- What do I find beautiful in my life?
- What helps me relax into a deep, peaceful, receptive state?
- What prevents me from listening to and acting upon my intuitive insights?
- Is there any work I need to do on my lower chakras in order to be able to work safely with and to reap the benefits of working with the third eye chakra?
- If my subconscious, and the Universal Conscious, were to give me a healing symbol, what would it be?

CHAPTER 11

Crown Chakra
(Sahasrara)

Discover the Power of Everyday Ecstasy

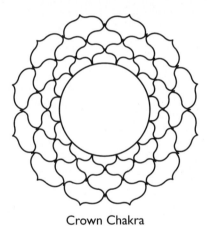

Crown Chakra

Working with this chakra is transformative, releasing your inner spark of genius and relaxing you into a state of pure bliss. You are now able to rise above everyday concerns and connect with the sacred. You are imbued with a sense of being at one with it all. You see the bigger picture and are no longer bogged down by the minutiae of life. You feel connected to the cosmos and open to receiving divine inspiration. You now can see the celestial within the commonplace. Dive deep and uncover your creative gold!

Crown Chakra at a Glance

Sanskrit Name: Sahasrara (thousand-spoked wheel)

Physical Location: Situated at or just above the crown of the head

Element: Consciousness

Colors: Violet, gold, white

Yantra: It is often depicted as a full moon–like circle.

Seed Mantra: Om

Affirmations: *The light of love surrounds me. Light of love within, light of love without. Light of love, guide me home.*

Main Creative Concerns: Seeing the bigger picture, putting aside ego, connecting to the divine mystery and channeling this cosmic awareness into your creativity.

Balanced: Fulfilled, imaginative, peaceful, inspired, inspirational, spiritual leader, sexually fulfilled and responsible, sees the bigger picture, insightful, open to blissful states, sense of connectedness, creative.

Excessive: Egotistical, superficial, spiritually arrogant, charlatan, false messiah, overzealous, sexually irresponsible, addictive personality, irrational, unworldly, flits from one craze to another convinced it will lead to enlightenment.

Deficient: Unimaginative, bland, detached, closed mind, aloof, unspiritual, materialistic, small-minded, tunnel vision, stuck in their ways, over-rational, takes things at face value, uninspired.

Life Issues: Finding fulfillment, seeking enlightenment, balancing spiritual and material concerns, sexuality, developing an ability to put self-interest aside and work for the greater good, acting from a place of love, awakening to a realization of the oneness of creation.

Healing Practices: Meditation, mantra, Tantric sexual practices, loving relationships, visualization, prayer, being in spiritual communion with others, mindfulness, compassion, self-compassion, yoga, random acts of kindness, yoga nidra, walking, being in nature, stargazing, creative pursuits, playing and listening to uplifting music, viewing inspirational art, creative collaboration with others, any work that is for the common good.

Cosmic Consciousness

The crown chakra is depicted as a thousand-petaled white lotus. It is here that Shakti is united with Shiva, and we rest in a state of pure bliss. The ancient yogis described this ecstatic state as one of unity. The smaller, ego self dissolves, and any sense of separation from the cosmos evaporates. All is one, and we are part of it all. We perceive ourselves as a miniscule but precious part of an infinite universe.

The creativity of the ancient yogis was on a truly cosmic scale. They turned their gaze inward and discovered mirrored within their own body the whole cosmos. Whereas this truth was revealed to the yogi through transcendent states of meditation, modern science now confirms that we are literally made of stardust!

Throughout the ages, yogis, shamans, mystics, and poets have traveled through the cosmos in their minds. And there are common themes that run through all their reports from their mystic travels. These include a sense of their ego-self dissolving into a boundless, loving presence and a feeling of coming home. Intriguingly, astronauts, looking down on Earth from space, also often describe "feeling at one with humanity, the Earth, or even the entire cosmos." They talk of a sense of there being something so much bigger than them, that dwarfs their own importance. Apollo 14's Edgar Mitchell, on his return journey from the moon, felt that the entire universe was "in some way conscious," and he said, "I was overwhelmed with the sensation of physically and mentally extending out into the cosmos."[36] Both poets, mystics, yogis, and astronauts share in common the experience of feeling unified with a cosmos that is itself an ensouled being.

Astronauts, of course, experience the ultimate shift in perspective when looking down on our planet Earth from space. And although most of us won't ever go into space, we can still experience that sense of awe and wonder down here on Earth. The crown chakra is associated with these transcendent states of pure bliss. When the crown chakra is awakened, we feel a sense of being at one with the world. Our sense of separation dissolves and we feel connected to all that is. The realm of the crown chakra is one of wonder and awe.

It is possible that you have already experienced a taste of this rapturous sense of union associated with the crown chakra. You might have experienced it while doing yoga, meditating, gardening, walking in nature, looking at the night sky, breastfeeding your baby, bathing in the ocean, making love, or when fully absorbed in a creative activity. Scientists

---

36. Jo Marchant, *The Human Cosmos: A Secret History of the Stars* (Edinburgh, UK: Canongate Books, 2020), 269–70.

are now discovering what poets and mystics have known for millennia: that experiencing awe and wonder has an enduringly positive impact on our health, well-being, and even our creativity.[37]

Awe is what we experience when we come face to face with the mystery that lies at the heart of the cosmos. Okay, so you and I might not be able to view Earth from space like an astronaut, but we can all gaze in wonder on a moonless night at the stars streaming out into infinity. We can also experience the divine mystery, like the ancient yogis, by tuning in to our crown chakra, our ego-self dissolving, as we relax into cosmic consciousness. This is the transcendent state of the crown chakra.

Channeling Cosmic Consciousness into Your Creations

All the work we have done so far on the lower chakras prepares us to experience the rapturous state of awe associated with the crown chakra. Studies have shown that experiencing states of awe promotes heightened creativity and open-mindedness.[38] Likewise, when we regularly connect with the awe-inspiring divine mystery through our chakra meditation practice, the positive effects are enduring and illuminate and inspire our creative process. The transcendent states of the crown chakra help us rise above our smaller, ego self and plug into a larger cosmic consciousness. We are bathed in light, and we channel this light and love into our creations. The singer becomes the song. The dancer merges with the dance. The poet is the pen that writes across the page. The sculptor merges with the stone that she is carving. The painter is the color splashed upon the canvas.

If you want your creativity to flourish, it's important to uncover what inspires you with a sense of awe and wonder. Virtuoso performances can inspire awe. Some of us feel it when we watch a superhuman sports achievement, stand in front of a sublime work of art, or hear a heavenly piece of music. Light pouring through a stained-glass window in a cathedral. Rodin's sculpture *The Kiss*. A waterfall, a canyon, the ocean, the Milky Way's river of stars stretching into infinity, moonlight on water. A child's smile. Holding your lover's hand. It pays to take time to discover what is awe-inspiring for you and to create opportunities to immerse yourself in that experience, whether it's visiting an art gallery, climbing a mountain, or spending time in meditation.

---

37. Marchant, *The Human Cosmos*, 266–67.

38. Alice Chirico et al., "Awe Enhances Creative Thinking: An Experimental Study," *Creativity Research Journal* 30, no. 2 (2018): 123–31, doi:10.1080/10400419.2018.1446491.

Another way of ensuring that your creativity taps into this awesome higher power is to live and work by your values. I find that my world shrinks when I am fearful or anxious, whereas it expands again when I remember my values and allow them to guide me, rather than being bullied by anxious thoughts. My values remind me of the bigger picture and that it's possible, even when I am anxious, to take valued actions and become the change I want to see in the world. Take time to clarify your values, let go of what you think they *should* be, and remember that they are unique to you and reflect your cares and concerns, which might be very different from those around you. Once you've established what your values are and started living your life in accordance with them, expect to be energized!

And finally, a character in Alice Walker's *The Color Purple* said, "I think it pisses God off if you walk by the color purple in a field somewhere and don't notice it."[39] Open your eyes and awaken to the awe-inspiring beauty of the world all around you. To do this is to open to the possibility of enlightenment in each and every moment, and in turn you can channel this everyday ecstasy into your creative process.

Yoga Inspired by the Crown Chakra

When we work with the crown chakra, it is important that we maintain an energetic connection with the lower chakras, particularly the root chakra, to ensure that we don't get too spaced out when working at this more spiritual, ethereal level. A physical yoga practice is the perfect way of staying grounded while you open yourself up to the blissful states of the crown chakra.

We can cultivate a meditative, prayerful quality to the practice by including slow, flowing yoga sequences (*vinyasas*), combining mantras with yoga asanas, and visualizing light circulating in and around the body. During periods of relaxation and meditation, we create the right conditions for the crown chakra to blossom.

Other practices that are conducive to working with the crown chakra are yoga nidra, guided visualizations, the *metta bhavana* (loving kindness meditation), repetition of the mantra *Om*, pranayama, partner yoga, and Tantric sexual practices within a loving relationship.

---

39. Alice Walker, *The Color Purple* (New York: Harcourt, 2003), 196.

Crown Chakra Yoga Practice

The aim of the practice is to develop an awareness of the crown chakra, and we prepare the ground for this by first focusing on the lower chakras to ensure stability. In the first part of the practice, we use standing poses for grounding, and this creates a sense of a journeying up through the chakras. We visualize light imagery and use mantras to give the practice a meditative and devotional feel.

The affirmation we use in the practice is *Love and light within. Love and light without.* We coordinate it with the breath in this way:

Inhale: Love and light within

Exhale: Love and light without

Allow 20 to 30 minutes.

At the end of these instructions, you'll find an illustrated aide-mémoire for the whole practice.

1. Crown Chakra Awareness Exercise

Find a comfortable seated position. Be aware of where your body is in contact with the floor and relax into the support of the earth beneath you.

Now, bring your awareness to the base of the spine and travel your awareness up through the spine to the crown of the head. Then maintain your awareness at the space just above the crown of the head and silently repeat the chakra's affirmation, coordinating it with the breath. Inhale and affirm, *Light of love within.* Exhale and affirm, *Light of love without.*

Crown Chakra Awareness Exercise

2. Mountain Pose (*Tadasana*)

Stand tall, feet parallel and about hip width apart. Be aware of the contact between your feet and the earth beneath you. Imagine a string attached to the crown of your head, gently pulling you skyward; simultaneously, let your tailbone drop and feel your heels rooting down into the earth.

Now, bring your awareness to your spine and imagine that the spine is a tall column bathed in light. Maintain this image of the spine as a column bathed in light throughout the practice.

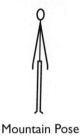

Mountain Pose

3. Bend and straighten warm-up

Take the legs 2 to 3 feet apart and turn the toes slightly out. Take the arms out to the sides at shoulder height, palms facing downward. On your next exhale, bend the knees and lower the arms. Inhaling, return to the starting position. You can silently coordinate the breath and movement with the affirmation. Inhale and affirm, *Love and light within.* Exhale and affirm, *Love and light without.* Repeat 8 times.

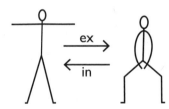

Bend and straighten warm-up

4. Warrior Flow (*Virabhadrasana Vinyasa*)

The following are steps for Warrior Flow (*Virabhadrasana Vinyasa*):

4a. Warrior 2 (*Virabhadrasana 2*)

To start this flowing sequence, take the legs 2 to 3 feet apart, turning the left foot slightly in and the right foot out. Bend the right knee. Take the arms out at shoulder height, palms facing down. Turn your head to look along your right arm. Stay here for a few breaths.

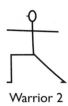

Warrior 2

4b. Reverse Warrior Pose (*Virabhadrasana* variation)

Keeping the right knee bent, lower the left hand to rest on the outside of the left thigh, reach the right arm up above the head and over to the left, and look up at the raised arm. Stay here for a few breaths.

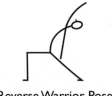

Reverse Warrior Pose

4c. Side-Angle Pose (*Utthita Parsvakonasana*)

Take the right forearm to rest on the right thigh (or for a stronger pose reach the hand down to the floor), taking the left arm over toward the left ear, and keep the chest rotating skyward. Stay here for a few breaths.

Repeat steps 4a, 4b, and 4c on the other side.

Side-Angle Pose

4d. Wide-Leg Standing Forward Bend (*Prasarita Padottanasana*)

The legs are 2 to 3 feet apart and the feet are parallel. Raise the arms out to the sides, just below shoulder height. Inhaling, hinge forward from the hip joints into a wide-leg forward bend. Bring the hands to the floor. For a gentler option bring the hands to rest on the legs or on raised blocks. Stay here for a few breaths, and then return to the starting position.

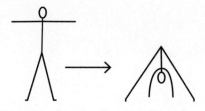

Wide-Leg Standing Forward Bend Pose

5. Dancer Pose (*Natarajasana*)

Stand tall, feet hip width apart and arms by your sides. Bend your right knee, and with your right hand catch hold of your ankle. Take the left arm up above the head. Then tip the torso forward, extending the back foot up and away from you and reaching forward and up with the opposite arm. Stay for a few breaths and then repeat on the other side. If you have balance problems, practice facing a wall, with your extended hand resting on the wall for support.

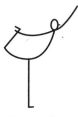

Dancer Pose

6. *Ram-Yam-Lam* Sequence

Stand tall, feet parallel and about hip-width apart, with hands resting on the solar plexus. Inhale and take the arms out to the sides. On the exhale, chant *Ram* (pronounced *rum*), as you bring your hands back to the solar plexus. Inhale, taking the arms overhead. Exhale, lowering the arms and crossing the hands to the heart as you chant *Yam* (pronounced *yum*). Inhale, taking the arms overhead. Exhale, coming into a Standing Forward Bend (*Uttanasana*), chanting *Lam* (pronounced *lum*). Inhale, come back up to standing, taking both arms up above the head. Exhale, lowering the hands back to the solar plexus. Repeat the sequence 3 more times.

Ram-Yam-Lam Sequence

7. Downward-Facing Dog Pose (*Adho Mukha Svanasana*) into Upward-Facing Dog Pose (*Urdhva Mukha Svanasana*)

Come in to Downward-Facing Dog Pose (*Adho Mukha Svanasana*). Inhale and swing into Upward-Facing Dog Pose (*Urdhva Mukha Svanasana*). Exhale back into Downward-Facing Dog Pose. As you alternate between these two poses, silently coordinate the breath and movement with the affirmation. Inhale and affirm, *Love and light within.* Exhale and affirm, *Love and light without.* Repeat 6 times.

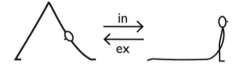

Downward-Facing Dog Pose into Upward-Facing Dog

8. Seated Twist (*Ardha Matsyendrasana*) variation

Come to a seated position, legs outstretched. Bend your right knee and place your right foot on the outside of your left knee. Sit up tall, wrap your left arm around your right knee and hug the knee into your chest. Place your right palm down on the floor behind you. Inhale, lengthen up through your spine, exhale, and twist, looking over your right shoulder.

During your stay in the twist, on each inhale, visualize your spine as a tall column, bathed in light. And on each exhale, drop your awareness down to your belly. Stay for a few breaths and then repeat on the other side. (More experienced students might wish to substitute a more complex seated twist here.)

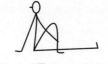

Seated Twist variation

9. Heart Chakra Sequence

Start in Child's Pose (*Balasana*), with forearms and hands on the floor, just above your head. Inhale and come up to tall kneeling, taking your arms above your head. Exhale, chanting the mantra *Yam* as you cross your hands and place them at your heart. Inhale, raising the arms above your head again. Exhale, coming back to Child's Pose. Repeat the sequence 6 times.

If you are pushed for time, end your practice here.

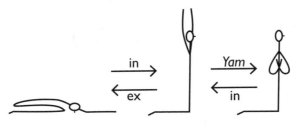

Heart Chakra Sequence

10. Crown Chakra Meditation

If you have more time, then come into a comfortable seated position for the Crown Chakra Meditation that follows the overview of this practice.

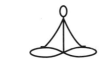

Crown Chakra Meditation

11. Mantra *Ma* and arm movements

After you work with the crown chakra, the mantra *Ma* is a wonderful way of grounding yourself, ready to resume your everyday activities.

In a seated position, rest your hands on your belly. Inhale and take your arms out to the side. Exhale and bring your hands back to the belly, chanting the mantra *Ma* (*mm-ah*).

Repeat 6 times.

Please note that in this exercise we divide the mantra *Ma* into two syllables, *mm* and *ah*. Making a prolonged *mm* sound, direct your awareness to the third eye chakra, between the brows, and making a prolonged *ah* sound, direct your awareness to the sacral chakra at the belly.

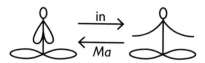

Mantra *Ma* and arm movements

Crown Chakra Yoga Practice Overview

1. Crown Chakra Awareness Exercise

2. Mountain Pose with column of light imagery

3. Bend and straighten warm-up × 8. Inhale: *Love and light within.* Exhale: *Love and light without.*

4. Warrior Flow

5. Dancer Pose

6. *Ram-Yam-Lam* Sequence × 4

7. Downward-Facing Dog Pose into Upward-Facing Dog Pose × 6. Inhale: *Love and light within.* Exhale: *Love and light without.*

8. Seated Twist variation with column of light imagery

9. Heart Chakra Sequence × 6. *End here if short of time.*

10. Crown Chakra Meditation

11. Mantra *Ma* and arm movements × 6

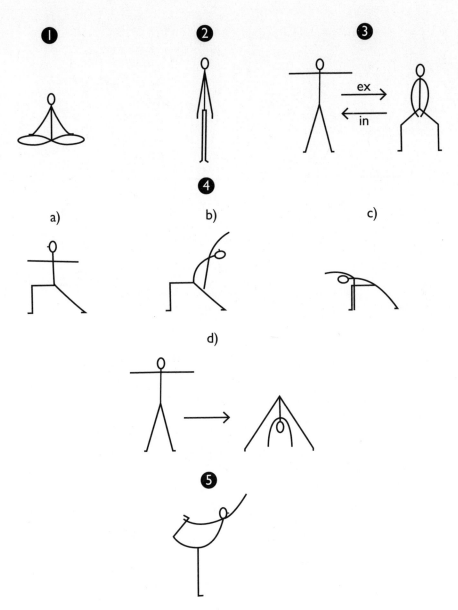

Crown Chakra Yoga Practice Overview

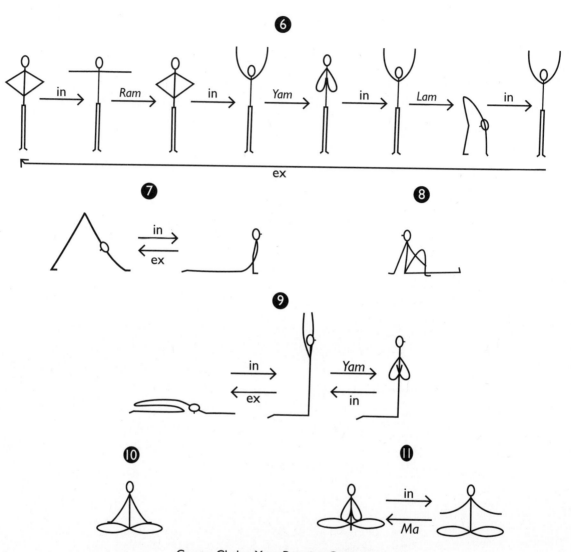

Crown Chakra Yoga Practice Overview

MEDITATION

Crown Chakra Meditation

This meditation can be used to begin or end a yoga practice, and it can also be used on its own as a standalone practice.

This meditation is gently energizing, is healing, and will help to lighten your mood. It creates the right conditions for you to connect with your cosmic consciousness and unfold into the blissful state associated with the crown chakra.

Find a comfortable seated or lying position. Be aware of where your body is in contact with the floor and relax into the support of the earth beneath you.

Now, bring your awareness to the base of the spine and travel your awareness up through the spine to the crown of the head. Then maintain your awareness at the space just above the crown of the head and silently repeat the chakra's affirmation, coordinating it with the breath:

Inhale: *Light of love within*

Exhale: *Light of love without*

Keeping your awareness at the space just above the crown of the head, picture a many-petaled white lotus flower, its petals opening to the sun. Visualize the two roots of the flower crisscrossing down the length of the spine and at the base of spine dividing into many roots that travel down from your body deep down into the earth below.

Now, picture a shaft of golden sunlight illuminating your flower and radiating rays of sunlight around your body. Luxuriate in the beauty of the lotus flower and allow yourself to relax into and enjoy the warm, healing light that surrounds you.

When you feel ready, let go of the image of the lotus flower. Notice how you are feeling now. Once again become aware of where your body is in contact with the earth beneath you.

If you are resuming your everyday activities after this meditation, then to conclude this meditation do the Chakra-Closing Lotus Visualization (see page 26).

MEDITATION

Crown Chakra Blissful Walking Meditation

In this walking meditation we are increasing our capacity for joy by honing our ability to find joy in a million small everyday experiences. You can do this meditation anywhere—in your house from room to room, in your garden, in a park, in the countryside, or in the town.

Begin the meditation by slightly slowing down your walking and becoming aware of the contact your feet are making with the earth with each step. Be aware of how your body feels as you walk and take joy in the act of walking. Maintain a gentle awareness of the natural flow of your breath.

As you walk, be on the lookout for anything that pleases you or that you find beautiful: dappled sunlight on the path, reflections of blue sky and clouds in a puddle, children playing, a squirrel darting up a tree. Be aware of any sensations that you feel: a breeze through your hair, warm sunlight on your face, drops of rain. Notice the aroma of cut grass or the scent of evergreen trees after rain. Listen to the sound of leaves rustling in the breeze, birds singing, raindrops on a tin roof. At the same time, be aware of anything that you find unpleasant—traffic fumes, cigarette smoke, a bitingly cold wind, and so on—but keep bringing your attention back to anything that you find pleasurable.

The crown chakra helps us cultivate a sense of being at one with the world. With this in mind, if you wish, you can begin to repeat an affirmation as you walk. The idea is to engender a feeling of unity with your surroundings. When you pass a tree, watch a cloud float by, stand by a river, see a bird of prey circling in the sky, or notice a passerby, then repeat the phrase *We are one*. Other phrases that you could use are *Thou art that* or *I am that* or *All in the circle of life*.

To conclude your walking meditation, return to noticing the contact your feet make with the earth with each step. Be aware of your breathing. Notice how you are feeling now. Try to take this sense of connection and unity into the next thing that you do today.

Crown Chakra Writing Meditation

For full instructions on how to do a writing meditation, go to the Writing Meditation with Focus section (see page 44).

Set your timer for 10 to 20 minutes and write meditatively on one or more of the following subjects:

- The light of love is…
- I am filled with awe and wonder when…
- When I live by my values, my fear shrinks and…
- Enlightenment is…
- Tantric sex

Crown Chakra Meditation Questions

For full instructions on how to use the meditation questions, see page 47.

- Which values are most important to me in my life and in my creativity?
- What helps me cultivate a sense of awe and wonder?
- Which art, literature, poetry, or other artform inspires and uplifts me?
- How can I introduce an awe-inspiring quality into my own work?
- How do I create the right conditions for everyday ecstasy to manifest in my life?

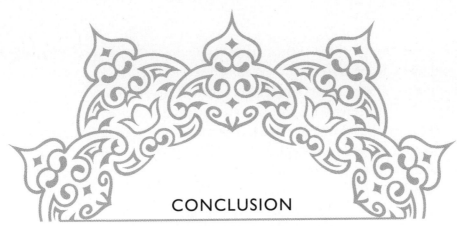

CONCLUSION

The Wheel Keeps on Turning

Congratulations, you have reached the end of the book and completed one turn around the wheel of the chakras! Our journey around the chakras is a circular rather than a linear one. The word chakra means "wheel," and its verbal root is *car*, "to move."[40] When we work with the chakras, we are moved, we are transformed, and we connect with a deep source of inspiration that nourishes our creative life. The circular nature of our journey around the chakras means that there is no endpoint. Every ending is a new beginning.

I hope that you will come to look upon this book as a good friend, returning to it whenever you feel in need of fresh inspiration. In time, as you become more experienced at working with the chakras, your inner wisdom will take over and let you know which chakra needs some extra attention. For example, if you are feeling anxious or unsupported, return to the root chakra chapter. If your creative work becomes all work and no pleasure, refer back to the sacral chakra chapter, which is also a good one for getting back into your creative ebb and flow. If you are in need of assertiveness, go to the solar

---

40. Feuerstein, *Encyclopedic Dictionary of Yoga*, 72.

plexus chakra chapter. If self-criticism is undermining your creative efforts, find some self-compassion in the heart chakra chapter. When you need to find your voice and speak up, the communication chakra chapter will empower you. The third eye chakra chapter will help you envisage what it is that you wish to create. The crown chakra chapter will plug you into cosmic consciousness, and when you're high on life, what can't you do?

Our challenge is to imbue our creations with the sense of awe and wonder that comes from working with the chakras. All the work we have done on the chakras will support us in this endeavor. The crown chakra unites us with our higher purpose. The third eye chakra inspires our vision, the communication chakra empowers our self-expression, the heart chakra ensures that our creations are imbued with love, the solar plexus chakra gives us the drive and determination to see our work through to completion, the sacral chakra gives us our creative ebb and flow and reminds us to move toward the pleasurable, and the root chakra nourishes and supports the roots of our lotus flower and creates the right conditions for our creativity to grow and blossom.

We live in a world that is a state of constant flux. Our spiritual progress tends to be similar to the childhood game of snakes and ladders. Just when we think we've reached the top, life tends to remind us with a slide down the snake that there's more work to be done lower down. Working with the chakras is a balancing act, and most of us will regularly need to revisit the lower chakras, associated with the material world, to check that we have strong enough foundations to support our work on the higher chakras. The Buddhist writer and teacher Jack Kornfield coined the phrase "after the ecstasy, the laundry" in his book of the same title, which is an insightful way to sum up the nature of our work on the chakras.[41] Enlightenment is not a final destination.

A mandala is a sacred circle used to represent the universe that serves as a tool for meditation. Buddhist monks spend days painstakingly constructing intricate sand mandalas. It takes a day for one monk to draw the mandala in chalk. After that, another monk, using a metal funnel, places millions of grains of brightly colored sand to make the intricately patterned mandala. He starts this process from the center and works concentrically outward. Once complete, a ceremony is held to bless the mandala. While the monks are chanting the blessing, one monk begins to destroy the mandala by dragging his knuckle through the sand. Another monk slowly and meditatively sweeps the sand from the perimeter to the center of the mandala with a paintbrush. Once the destruction of the mandala is complete, the monks sweep the sand and place it in an urn, then

---

41. Jack Kornfield, *After the Ecstasy, the Laundry* (London: Ebury Publishing, 2000).

pouring into flowing water as a way of giving back to the earth and bringing healing to the world.[42]

The creation and destruction of the sand mandala is a wonderful example of doing the work and letting go of the outcome. The monks prayerfully create something of exquisite beauty and then they let it go. For many of us our creations are like our babies, and it's hard to let them go and allow them to find their own way in the world. And, although we might not wish to scrape a knuckle through the sand of our creation, however, once we have created a book, or a painting, or other creation, we must cultivate the wisdom to know when it's the right time to release it, like a seed head on the wind, and trust that it will land on fertile ground. I hope that the practices in this book have equipped you with the skills to enjoy and be fully present to the creative process from conception through to bringing it out into the light of the world.

Take a moment now, as you reach the end of this book, to pause … breathe in, breathe out, pause … relax … and then let the in-breath inspire you again. Life is a circle and within the circle is the Tree of Life. Your spine is a tree at the center of the world, its roots are in the earth, and its branches stretch up to the heavens. Along the central axis of the spine are seven flowers, and as each chakra's flower opens, you blossom into your full creative potential.

---

42. "Sacred Mandala," BBC, last modified November 23, 2009, https://www.bbc.co.uk/religion/religions/buddhism/customs/mandala.shtml.

Bibliography

Anh-Huong, Nguyen, and Thich Nhat Hanh. *Walking Meditation.* Boulder, CO: Sounds True, 2006.

Brown, Laura S. *Your Turn for Care: Surviving the Aging and Death of the Adults Who Harmed You.* Self-published, 2012.

Budilovsky, Joan, and Eve Adamson. *The Complete Idiot's Guide to Yoga.* Indianapolis, IN: Alpha Books, 2001.

Chirico, Alice, Vlad Petre Glaveanu, Pietro Cipresso, and Giuseppe Riva. "Awe Enhances Creative Thinking: An Experimental Study." *Creativity Research Journal* 30, no. 2 (2018): 123–31. doi:10.1080/10400419.2018.1446491.

Desikachar, T. K. V. *The Heart of Yoga.* Rochester, VT: Inner Traditions, 1995.

Feuerstein, Georg. *Encyclopedic Dictionary of Yoga.* New York: Paragon House, 1990.

———. *The Yoga Tradition: Its History, Literature, Philosophy and Practice* Prescott, AZ: Hohm Press, 2001.

Hutchison Murray, William. *The Scottish Himalayan Expedition.* London: J. M. Dent & Sons, 1951.

Iyengar, B. K. S. *The Tree of Yoga.* London: Thorsons, 2000.

Kennerley, Helen. *Overcoming Childhood Trauma: A Self-Help Guide Using Cognitive Behavioural Techniques.* London: Constable & Robinson, 2009.

Kerouac, Jack. "Belief and Technique for Modern Prose." *Evergreen Review* 2, no. 8 (spring 1959): 57.

Kornfield, Jack. *After the Ecstasy, the Laundry.* London: Ebury Publishing, 2000.

Lerner, Harriet. *The Dance of Anger: A Woman's Guide to Changing the Patterns of Intimate Relationships.* London: HarperCollins UK, 2004.

Lusk, Julie. *Yoga Nidra Meditations: 24 Scripts for True Relaxation.* Woodbury, MN: Llewellyn Publications, 2021.

Marchant, Jo. *The Human Cosmos: A Secret History of the Stars.* Edinburgh, UK: Canongate Books, 2020.

Mascaro, Juan, trans. *The Upanishads.* London: Penguin, 1965.

Nhat Hanh, Thich. *Reconciliation: Healing the Inner Child.* Berkeley, CA: Parallax Press, California, 2010.

Nietzsche, Friedrich. *Twilight of the Idols and the Antichrist.* Translated by Thomas Common. Mineola, NY: Dover, 2004.

O'Mara, Shane. *In Praise of Walking.* London: Penguin Random House, 2019.

Stoler Miller, Barbara, trans. *Yoga: Discipline of Freedom; The Yoga Sutra Attributed to Patanjali.* New York: Bantam Books, 1998.

Walker, Alice. *The Color Purple.* New York: Harcourt, 2003.

———. *The World Has Changed: Conversations with Alice Walker.* Edited by Rudolph P. Byrd. New York: The New Press, 2010.

Walker, Barbara G. *The Woman's Dictionary of Symbols and Sacred Objects.* New York: HarperCollins, 1988.

———. *The Woman's Encyclopedia of Myths and Secrets.* New York: HarperCollins, 1983.

Recommended Resources

The Chakras

Eliade, Mircea. *Yoga: Immortality and Freedom*. Princeton, NJ: Princeton University Press, 1990.

Feuerstein, Georg. *The Yoga Tradition*. Prescott, AZ: Hohm Press, 2001.

Hall, Doriel. *Healing with Meditation*. Dublin: Gill & Macmillan, 1996.

Judith, Anodea. *Chakra Yoga*. Woodbury, MN: Llewellyn Publications, 2015.

———. *Eastern Body, Western Mind*. Berkeley, CA: Crown Publishing Group, 2004.

Kraftsow, Gary. *Yoga for Transformation*. New York: Penguin, 2002.

Simpson, Liz. *The Book of Chakra Healing*. London: Gaia Books, 1999.

Wills, Pauline. *Chakra Workbook: Rebalance Your Body's Vital Energy*. Dublin: Gill & Macmillan, 2002.

Creativity

Cameron, Julia. *The Artist's Way: A Course in Discovering and Recovering Your Creative Self*. London: Macmillan, 1995.

Éstes, Clarissa Pinkola. *Women Who Run With the Wolves: Contacting the Power of the Wild Woman*. London: Random House, 1998.

Kaufman, Scott Barry, and Carolyn Gregoire. *Wired to Create: Discover the 10 Things Great Artists, Writers, and Innovators Do Differently*. London: Ebury Publishing, 2015.

Walking Meditation

Anh-Huong, Nguyen, and Thich Nhat Hanh. *Walking Meditation*. Boulder, CO: Sounds True, 2006.

Nhat Hanh, Thich. *How to Walk*. Berkeley, CA: Parallax Press, 2015.

———. *The Long Road Turns to Joy: A Guide to Walking Meditation*. Berkeley, CA: Parallax Press, 1996.

Salzberg, Sharon, and Joseph Goldstein. *Insight Meditation Workbook*. Boulder, CO: Sounds True, 2001.

Mindfulness Meditation

Gilbert, Paul. *The Compassionate Mind*. London: Constable & Robinson, 2009.

Nhat Hanh, Thich. *Mindful Movements: Ten Exercises for Well-Being*. Berkeley, CA: Parallax Press, 2008.

Orsillo, Susan M., and Lizabeth Roemer. *The Mindful Way through Anxiety: Break Free from Chronic Anxiety and Reclaim Your Life*. New York: Guildford Press, 2011.

Williams, Mark, and Danny Penman. *Mindfulness: A Practical Guide to Finding Peace in a Frantic World*. London: Piatkus, 2011.

Writing and Writing Meditation

Goldberg, Natalie. *Writing Down the Bones: Freeing the Writer Within*. Boston, MA: Shambala Publications, 1986.

Magrs, Paul, and Julia Bell, eds. *The Creative Writing Coursebook*. London: Macmillan, 2001.

Rentzenbrink, Cathy. *Write It All Down: How to Put Your Life on the Page*. London: Macmillan, 2022.

The National Centre for Writing (affiliated to the University of East Anglia) offers creative writing courses to suit all levels and abilities and even some short free courses. Their online courses can be done from anywhere in the world and are a wonderful way of finding a writing community. Check out their website to find great resources and writerly tips: https://courses.nationalcenterforwriting.org.uk/.

Yoga Practice

There are so many brilliant resources for beginners and more experienced students to be found online, so explore and see what's out there and what appeals to you. Also, ask yoga friends for recommendations too. Below are some websites that I regularly use. Esther Ekhart's website is an invaluable resource for beginners and more experienced students.

www.yogajournal.com

www.ekhartyoga.com

There are so many wonderful yoga books available. Go online or to your local bookshop and see what appeals to you. The following are some of my favorite yoga books.

Bennett, Bija. *Emotional Yoga: How the Body Can Heal the Mind.* London, UK: Bantam Books, 2002.

Farhi, Donna. *Yoga Mind, Body & Spirit: A Return to Wholeness.* New York: Henry Holt, 2000.

Gates, Janice. *Yogini: The Power of Women in Yoga.* San Rafael, CA: Mandala Publishing, 2006.

Hall, Jean. *Breathe: Simple Breathing Techniques for a Calmer, Happier Life.* London: Quadrille Publishing, 2016.

Kraftsow, Gary. *Yoga for Wellness: Healing with the Timeless Teachings of Viniyoga.* New York: Penguin, 1999.

Lasater, Judith. *30 Essential Yoga Poses: For Beginning Students and Their Teachers*, Berkeley, CA: Rodmell Press, 2003.

———. *Living Your Yoga: Finding the Spiritual in Everyday Life.* Berkeley, CA: Rodmell Press, 2000.

Lee, Cyndi. *Yoga Body, Buddha Mind.* New York: Riverhead Books, 2004.

Powers, Sarah. *Insight Yoga.* Boston, MA: Shambhala Publications, 2008.

Rountree, Sage. *Everyday Yoga.* Boulder, CO: Velo Press, 2015.

Sabatini, Sandra. *Breath: The Essence of Yoga; A Guide to Inner Stillness.* London, UK: Thorsons, 2000.

Scaravelli, Vanda. *Awakening the Spine: The Stress-Free New Yoga That Works with the Body to Restore Health, Vitality, and Energy.* New York: HarperCollins, 1991.

To Write to the Author

If you wish to contact the author or would like more information about this book, please write to the author in care of Llewellyn Worldwide Ltd. and we will forward your request. Both the author and the publisher appreciate hearing from you and learning of your enjoyment of this book and how it has helped you. Llewellyn Worldwide Ltd. cannot guarantee that every letter written to the author can be answered, but all will be forwarded. Please write to:

Jilly Shipway
℅ Llewellyn Worldwide
2143 Wooddale Drive
Woodbury, MN 55125-2989
Please enclose a self-addressed stamped envelope for reply,
or $1.00 to cover costs. If outside the U.S.A., enclose
an international postal reply coupon.

Many of Llewellyn's authors have websites with additional information and resources. For more information, please visit our website at http://www.llewellyn.com.